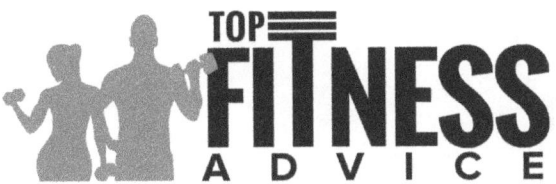

17-DAY SLIM DOWN

3rd Edition

Weight Loss Plan & Workouts For Flat Abs, Firm Butt & Lean Legs

LINDA WESTWOOD

First published in 2015 by Venture Ink Publishing

Copyright © Top Fitness Advice 2019

All rights reserved.

No part of this book may be reproduced in any form without permission in writing from the author. No part of this publication may be reproduced or transmitted in any form or by any means, mechanic, electronic, photocopying, recording, by any storage or retrieval system, or transmitted by email without the permission in writing from the author and publisher.

Requests to the publisher for permission should be addressed to publishing@ventureink.co

For more information about the contents of this book or questions to the author, please contact Linda Westwood at linda@topfitnessadvice.com

Disclaimer

This book provides wellness management information in an informative and educational manner only, with information that is general in nature and that is not specific to you, the reader. The contents of this book are intended to assist you and other readers in your personal wellness efforts. Consult your physician regarding the applicability of any information provided in this book to you.

Nothing in this book should be construed as personal advice or diagnosis, and must not be used in this manner. The information provided about conditions is general in nature. This information does not cover all possible uses, actions, precautions, side-effects, or interactions of medicines, or medical procedures. The information in this book should not be considered as complete and does not cover all diseases, ailments, physical conditions, or their treatment.

You should consult with your physician before beginning any exercise, weight loss, or health care program. This book should not be used in place of a call or visit to a competent health-care professional. You should consult a health care professional before adopting any of the suggestions in this book or before drawing inferences from it.

Any decision regarding treatment and medication for your condition should be made with the advice and consultation of a qualified health care professional. If you have, or suspect you have, a health-care problem, then you should immediately contact a qualified health care professional for treatment.

No Warranties: The author and publisher don't guarantee or warrant the quality, accuracy, completeness, timeliness, appropriateness or suitability of the information in this book, or of any product or services referenced in this book.

The information in this book is provided on an "as is" basis and the author and publisher make no representations or warranties of any kind with respect to this information. This book may contain inaccuracies, typographical errors, or other errors.

Liability Disclaimer: The publisher, author, and other parties involved in the creation, production, provision of information, or delivery of this book specifically disclaim any responsibility, and shall not be held liable for any damages, claims, injuries, losses, liabilities, costs, or obligations including any direct, indirect, special, incidental, or consequences damages (collectively known as "Damages") whatsoever and howsoever caused, arising out of, or in connection with the use or misuse of the site and the information contained within it, whether such Damages arise in contract, tort, negligence, equity, statute law, or by way of other legal theory.

Table of Contents

Disclaimer	3
Who is this book for?	9
What will this book teach you?	11
Introduction	13
Chapter 1: Transform Your Body in 17 Days	15
Chapter 2: Get Ready for the 17-Day Slim Down	23
Chapter 3: Let's Begin!	29
Chapter 4: Shed Those Pounds	33
Chapter 5: Get YOUR Flat Abs	39
Chapter 6: Firm Up Your Butt	47
Chapter 7: Want Lean Legs?	53
Chapter 8: The VITAL Ingredient to Weight Loss	61
Chapter 9: Breakfast Options	71
Chapter 10: Lunch Options	107
Chapter 11: Dinner Options	145
Chapter 12: Snacking Options	189
Chapter 13: Accelerate the Weight Loss	193
Chapter 14: After the 17 Days…	197
Chapter 15: Shopping List	201

Conclusion 213

Final Words 215

Would you prefer to listen to my book, rather than read it?

Download the audiobook version for free!

If you go to the special link below and sign up to Audible as a new customer, you can get the audiobook version of my book completely free.

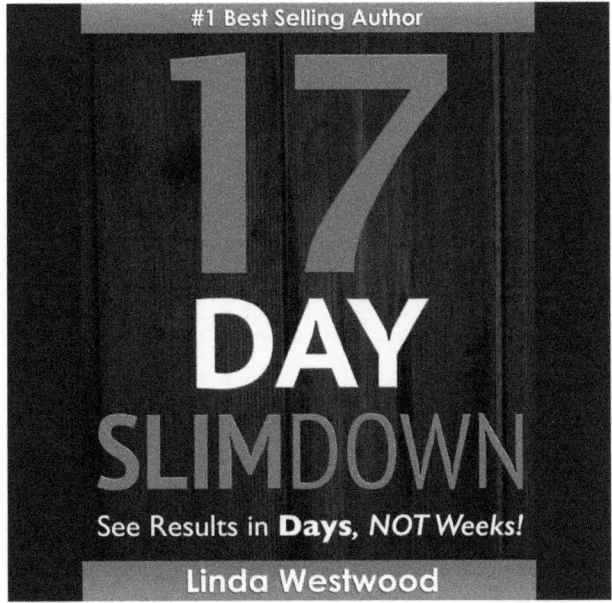

Go here to get your audiobook version for free:

TopFitnessAdvice.com/go/17day

Who is this book for?

Do you need a *strong* kick-start with your weight loss?

Are you ready for a full body transformation in just 17 days?

Do you just wish that your fat would just fall off *effortlessly?*

If you answered "Yes" to any of those questions – **this book is for you!**

I am going to share with you the most effective way to slim down and get flat abs, a firm butt and lean legs in just 17 days!

I have put it all together in this awesome 17-Day Slim Down plan!

The best part about is that you are going to see amazing results and this will *TRANSFORM YOUR BODY IN LESS THAN 3 WEEKS*!

You can be a complete beginner or someone who works out regularly, it doesn't matter!

If this sounds like it could help you, then keep reading...

What will this book teach you?

Inside, I will teach you one of the best ways to transform your body, especially your belly, butt and legs, which will not only boost your weight loss, but also rejuvenate both your mind and body!

You will feel the healthiest you have ever felt – have the most energy you have ever had – and the fat will be melting *constantly!*

How? Because you're going to be eating well, and doing some of the most effective workouts that accelerates body transformation in a short period of time.

In this book, I give you the plan right in front of you that will change your life – all you have to do is follow it!

One of the most important things for you to realize when reading this book is that this 17-Day Slim Down *really does work!*

However...

For you to achieve *real success*, you HAVE to apply this to your life.

This is where most people fail – they read through the entire book but do nothing. You MUST try your best to apply as you read through the book!

Introduction

I am delighted to introduce the 17-Day Slim Down, one of the most effective ways to lose weight – and keep it off for good.

During our busy modern lives, many of us slide into bad eating habits. It is hardly surprising – we are a time-poor society, always rushing around and grabbing fatty, snacks on the go, or quickly cooking high-calorie, over-processed ready meals.

This can become a way of life and then... well, it is no wonder that so many of us pile on the weight.

So how do we tackle our weight problems? All too often we turn to weird and wonderful 'solutions', the sort of faddy diets that involve us eating nothing but cabbage soup, for example.

Most of these crazy, unsustainable diets fail – we may lose a little weight if we manage to stick to their unrealistic rules, but we will actually wind up malnourished and cranky.

So cranky, in fact that we reach straight for the cookie jar again...

Time to choose a healthier path.

The 17-Day Slim Down is just that – a diet that is based on sensible eating principles, to give you everything you need in terms of protein, fiber, carbohydrates and a little healthy fat, whilst cutting out all of the junk.

It is a totally healthy way to eat, so much so that you could happily continue to eat along these lines for the rest of your life!

That's part one.

The other key part of the 17-Day Slim Down is the exercise factor. Those busy lives of us also, somehow, keep many of us spending more sedentary time that ever before.

Strangely, although we have little free time, we appear to mostly be busy driving everywhere, fiddling with our smartphones or sending emails... everything you can do sitting down. So our waists get thicker, our legs heavier and our behinds get out of shape – hardly surprising when you think about it.

Yet despite all this, most of us want trim, toned, healthy and attractive bodies. So, during the 17 days you will also do that vital part of any weight loss program - moving around!

This weight loss program includes some clearly defined daily exercises, which really will make a difference to the appearance of your body.

Are you getting excited? You should be – the next 17 days will involve you eating some of the best, healthiest foods of your life, plus exercising your way to a great new shape.

You will feel brighter, tighter and much lighter... so what are you waiting for?

Chapter 1

Transform Your Body in 17 Days

Welcome to the start of a 17-day phase that will transform your body, improve your health and potentially kick-start a whole new slim and fit episode of your life.

Many of us try hard to find the perfect weight loss program. Modern busy lives do not always allow for the preparation of complex dishes and yet few of us have a private chef to balance out the calories and nutrients in our diet!

As for exercise, few of us have the free time to indulge in a 3-hour workout, but we still long for a toned, slender physique...

The answer?

A slimming plan that offers a variety of easy-to-prepare meals and a manageable, enjoyable and effective exercise regime—the 17-Day Slim Down!

What is the 17-Day Slim Down?

The 17-Day Slim Down is an easy-to-follow weight loss program that really works. It incorporates a super-healthy diet and optimum levels of exercise, meaning that if you follow it to the letter you *WILL* see a fantastic difference – after just 17 days.

When you follow the 17-Day Slim Down you will not only enjoy seeing the pounds melt away, you will also be able to tone up your body so that it looks better than ever.

Why does it work?

This weight loss program works brilliantly because it focuses on filling you up with low-calorie, high-fiber, nutritious food and working your body in all the right places, resulting in you losing the pounds and getting closer to that great-looking body you have always wanted.

It is not a crash diet; it is not based on any weird dietary principles.

It is a foolproof way to shed excess weight and tone up, based on what the best nutritionists and personal trainers tell us – eat less, move more.

Do this for 17 days and you will not fail to see fabulous improvements, both on the scales and in the mirror.

You will feel great too!

During the 17-Day Slim Down you will:

- Eat breakfast, lunch, dinner and a snack every day, chosen from the 17 options for each meal.

- Drink a lot of water and/or unsweetened herbal tea.

- Exercise regularly in 17-minute workouts, enjoying both cardio and toning exercises that will work wonders for your abs, butt and legs.

How does the 17-Day Slim Down work?

The 17-Day Slim Down works along the lines of a few simple but highly effective principles:

- **Low-calorie, high-fiber food** – All of the recipes in the book contain plenty of fresh fruit and vegetables, healthy lean meats, fish and other protein, plenty of whole grains and minimally processed ingredients.

    As they fill you up, help your digestion work at its best and provide lots of essential nutrients for very few calories, they really are a recipe for total success!

- **Avoiding bloating foods** – Certain foods want work against your digestive system and irritate it or make it sluggish, often causing bloating.

    The 17-Day Slim Down recipes eliminate foods that are known to commonly cause bloating, so that you feel comfortable and so your internal engine continues to run at the optimum speed for burning those calories.

- **Daily cardio** – Rev up that engine and burn even more calories – it's that simple. Many people avoid daily exercise because they do not have the time energy or inclination to jump around for an hour or two.

Just the thought of so much exercise can be intimidating and off-putting. But how about 17 minutes of exercise?

This is a much more manageable slice of time and something that anyone can manage, which is why this program is so successful.

- **Effective, targeted toning exercise** – On top of the cardio, this weight loss plan incorporates 17 minutes of great exercises that will help you lose weight, flatten your belly, tone up your legs and beautifully firm your butt - perfect!

After the slim down, we will lead you forward into maintaining a much healthier new lifestyle that you can sustain, all clearly outlined in Chapter 14.

For now, let's just focus on getting ready to lose weight and discover a slimmer new you at last.

Discover Scientifically-Proven "Shortcuts" & "Hacks" to Lose Weight FASTER (With Very Little Effort)

For this month only, you can get Linda's best-selling & most popular book absolutely free – *Weight Loss Secrets You NEED to Know.*

Get Your FREE Copy Here:

TopFitnessAdvice.com/Bonus

Discover scientifically-proven tips to help you lose weight faster and easier than ever before. With this book, readers were able to improve their weight loss results and fitness levels. So, it's highly recommended that you get this book, especially while it's free!

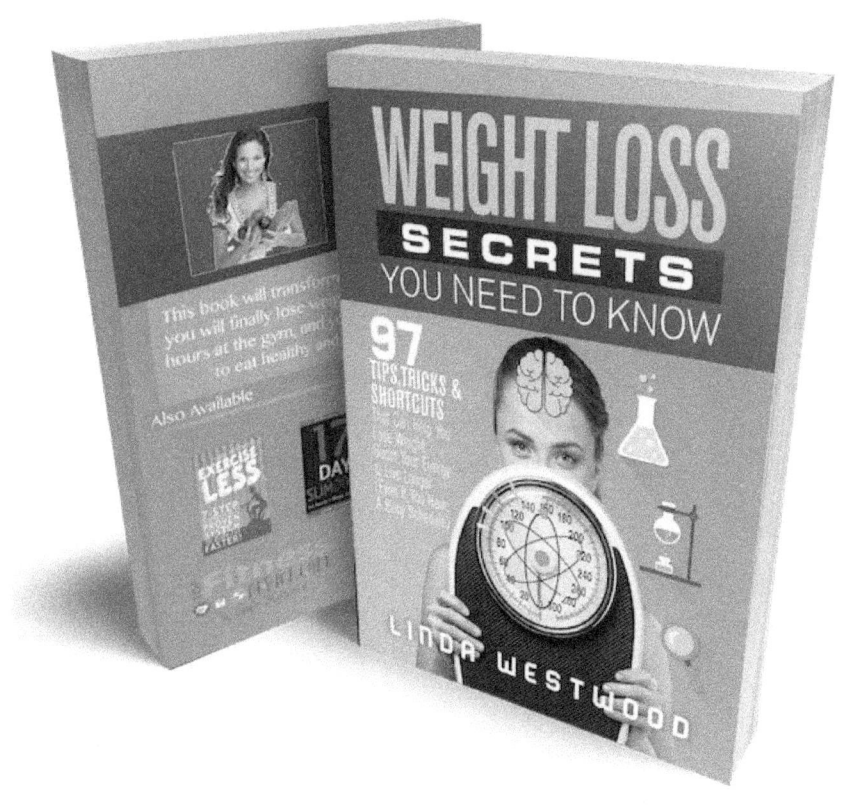

Get Your FREE Copy Here:

TopFitnessAdvice.com/Bonus

Chapter 2

Get Ready for the 17-Day Slim Down

Okay, time to prepare to change your life!

There are a few simple and fun steps that you should take before embarking on the 17-Day Slim Down. Do not be tempted to skip these steps as they will encourage you and make the whole process far more enjoyable plus they will help you measure the success of the program.

If you follow through all of these steps then you are going to guarantee your best chances of success on this diet.

Don't worry, there are only 3 steps for preparation.

Step 1 – Get in the right mindset

A little mental preparation at this stage can make all the difference. Time think positive and quash any residual doubts. How? Get a pen and paper and write down your own answers to these questions:

1. Why am I going on this 17-Day Slim Down?

2. What are the potential pitfalls that I must avoid?

3. What is my number one aim through doing this program?

Answer these questions and clarify for yourself why you are going to follow the program.

As a final tip, check-off some of the many benefits of losing weight:

- Look better than you have done in years – younger, fitter and more attractive.
- Drastically cut your risk of cancer, heart disease, stroke, diabetes and other potentially fatal diseases.
- Enjoy fitting into your favorite smaller-size clothes again, or treating yourself to new ones – it is a real ego boost!
- Feel more energetic and able to enjoy more activities.
- Eliminate toxins from your system with a high-fiber, high-water diet.
- Enjoy glowing skin and improve your complexion.
- Benefit from improved digestion – you may find that any internal issues you have been having simply melt away.

Step 2 – Doing the 'before' body prep

Thinking about your body shape and vital statistics before you begin will provide inspiration throughout the 17 days:

Measure Up

Fun time! Take some measurements of your body before you begin. Then keep a record of them and see how you measure up after the 17 days.

Simply take a tape measure and record the size of various areas of your body – you can keep a record of them here:

BEFORE:

Waist _____

Hips _____

Thighs _____

Calves _____

Upper arms _____

AFTER:

Waist _____

Hips _____

Thighs _____

Calves _____

Upper arms_____

Take a Before and After Selfie

Stay motivated throughout the program by taking a photograph of yourself at the start of the program.

Be honest (ditch the make-up and make sure it shows you in its full natural glory, when you may be looking and feeling and bit overweight, pasty and blurred around the edges).

Then, simply look forward taking another photo after the 17-Day Slim Down. You may be amazed at the difference in your appearance – a slimmer profile and a wonderful glow.

Dig Out those 'Skinny Jeans'

It is vital to keep your aims at the forefront of your mind when you are losing weight.

Open your wardrobe and unearth a piece of clothing that you want to be able to get into and hang it on the wardrobe door for a moment.

Wouldn't you look great – if you could just get into it?

Stay on track and soon you'll be wearing it!

Step 3 – Get Ready to Shop!

Nutrition is the most essential part of weight loss, period. This book provides you with a wide range of recipes that will have you feeling slim, happy and healthy in 17 days.

The recipes are simple and you can stock up as you go along – there is even a comprehensive shopping list and store-cupboard check-list.

Just choose your recipes, or opt to try every single one over 17 days if you prefer. Then, turn to Chapter 15, select the ingredients that you need and go shop!

Chapter 3

Let's Begin!

Great – it is time to get started!

To keep things really simple, here's a clear breakdown of what you need to do over the next 17 days.

1. **Choose your meals**

   There are 17 meals for breakfast, 17 lunches, 17 dinners and 17 once-a-day snack options. Simply pick a different one each day and work through all of them, or select your favorites and stick to those – whatever you find easiest.

   Of course, if you find that one or more of the dishes are not to your taste, don't worry at all.

   Simply eat another one of the recipes or even substitute it for one of your own favorites. You just have to remember to keep it low in calories and high in fiber with a focus on fresh foods and wholegrains.

2. **Exercise is a very important part of the 17-Day Slim Down**

   Not everyone feels that they are well suited to exercise, but it is amazing how you can enjoy and benefit from just a few minutes every day.

In every area of the 17-Day Slim Down, 17 is the magic number!

In order to maximize your weight loss, you will therefore do 17 minutes of exercise, every morning and every evening, for 17 days.

Embrace it – you will feel great!

3. **This means that every morning, you will do 17 minutes of cardio**

In the next chapter we will look into the benefits that regular
cardio offers and the various types of cardio that you can enjoy.

4. **Every evening, you will carry out the body transformation toning exercises**

These will give you a flatter stomach with more defined abs, better, more slender legs and a firmer, more toned butt.

Again, each set of exercise that you do will only take 17 minutes.

5. **You will rotate the toning exercises so that each part of your body – abs, legs, or butt - only gets exercised once every three days**

These rotations are crucial as they will ensure that the correct muscles are rested enough and can ultimately perform better, helping you to slim down.

To find out more about the exercises that will get you into shape over the next 17 days – read on...

I hope that you are enjoying this book so far, and if you could spare 30 seconds, I would greatly appreciate you leaving a review on Amazon.com.

Chapter 4

Shed Those Pounds

Time to start moving more and getting rid of those excess pounds.

Carrying extra weight can make us look and feel less than our best, plus it is very bad for our health. Some leading doctors have claimed that if we could see how the unwanted fat was hampering our vital organs, we would act much more urgently.

Do you want to wait until you are ill? Of course not. Let's make a change, starting now.

Exercise is a key part of that change and this program has a simple regime to follow.

First comes the cardio, which you will carry out every morning. But what exactly will it do for you?

What is cardio?

Cardio is short for cardiovascular, which indicates that it is good for getting your heart going.

Also known as aerobic exercise, cardio really gets you moving about and really gets you out of breath as it is designed to get more oxygen into your blood.

Sound worrying? Not at all!

When you start to puff, your body will also be sending a load of feel-good hormones called endorphins around your body and serotonin will be creating a sweet natural buzz in your brain. This is genuinely exercise as pleasure, not pain.

In any case, it only last 17 minutes!

Which exercise to choose

There are endless cardio exercises to choose from. It does not have to be just running (although if you love it, do it), it can be any number of fun activities.

The only rule is – if it gets you moving, and healthily out of breath, then go for it!

Here are some cardio exercise ideas, which are great fun, will get you moving, and which you can do in the morning for a burst of 17 minutes:

- Adult gymnastics to music
- Aerobics workout, medium to high energy
- Aqua aerobics, medium to fast-paced
- Capoeira
- Cycling
- Disco dancing, vigorous
- Flamenco dancing
- Hiking at a good pace in the great outdoors
- Hula hooping
- Ice skating, medium to fast
- Jazz dancing
- Just Dance computer game

- Kick-boxing home workout
- Nordic Walking, vigorous
- Off-road mountain biking
- Rollerblading
- Running
- Salsa
- Skipping
- Swimming
- Tap-dancing, energetic
- Tango
- Trampolining
- Ultimate Frisbee
- Urban dance
- Walking, at least 3 mph
- Wii Tennis, Wii Fit etc
- Zumba

So – just how much can you get done in only 17 minutes?

The answer is... plenty!

You don't need hours to make an impact on your body. Make life easy for yourself, get your smartphone and set the time to exactly 17 minutes and then just get going...

Take a look at these sample cardio workouts based on the exercise options above and you will see how easily the 17 minutes can just fly by!

Example 1 – Interval Training... in Just 17 Minutes

This is easier when done to music, so turn up your best tunes loud – you might feel less inhibited if no one else is around!

Warm up by marching on the spot, lifting the legs high for one minute.

Follow up with 10 jumping jacks, then drop and do a plank for 30 seconds. Repeat x2.

Lift your right knee and bring your left elbow down to meet it, then swap sides – do this 20 times.

Reach up to the sky and lift your knees as if you are climbing a rope for 30 seconds. Then drop and do a plank for 30 seconds. Repeat x3.

Touch one foot with the opposite hand 20 times. Repeat x3.

Do the box-step. Step left foot, then right foot forward, raising the corresponding arm. Then put your left foot and right foot back and lower the matching arm. Do this vigorously 15 times over.

Go for a brisk walk, even if it is just around your own house. Swing your arms and take enthusiastic strides – if you have stairs to go up and down, this is even better. Do this for 5 minutes – make sure you keep moving.

Return to your original spot and do 10 more jumping jacks.

Now do the Grapevine. Stride sideways, crossing your steps and your arms as you scissor – 5 steps left then 5 steps right. Touch your toes, reach to the sky and then repeat x4.

Stretch up to the ceiling as high as you can, then slowly bend from the waist to touch your toes. Uncurl your spine very slowly until you are upright again, then stop.

You're done!

Example 2: Simple Swimming... for 17 minutes!

These exercises are based on a 25-meter length pool, as not everyone is lucky enough to live within a short distance of an Olympic-sized pool of 50 meters.

Get into the water at the shallow end and start doing the front crawl. Do 5 laps. Now it's time to do some water-running. Stand on the floor of the pool and run as fast as you can towards the other end. The water resistance will slow you right down, but keep going.

When you are starting to get out of your depth, turn around and run back in the other direction. Keep water-running for a full 5 minutes, ending up back at the shallow end.

Now do the back crawl for 5 laps; next do a final front crawl for 5 laps.

If you are super-fast and have a minute or two left to spare, do some gentle stretching exercise against the wall.

Then – your time is up!

Example 3 – Disco Dancing... for 17 Minutes!

This cardio is the easiest of the lot, as it will inevitably be done in your own inimitable style.

The instructions are very simple.

Put on your favorite pop music, nice and loud. Then – dance!

Wave those arms, move those feet and shake that booty without stopping for 17 minutes... and that's it!

Do any of these exercises and you will feel refreshed, younger, fitter and healthily worn out, which means you have burnt some serious calories.

Not a bad pay-off for just 17 minutes of exercise.

Chapter 5

Get YOUR Flat Abs

Super-trim and flat abs are many dieters' dream – but how do you achieve them? The answer is simple.

In conjunction with the foolproof weight loss food plan, you need to do some toning exercises to transform your body. Remember to do these in the evening for 17 minutes, once every three days (between your thigh and butt workouts).

Here's how to flatten those abs:

Super Eights

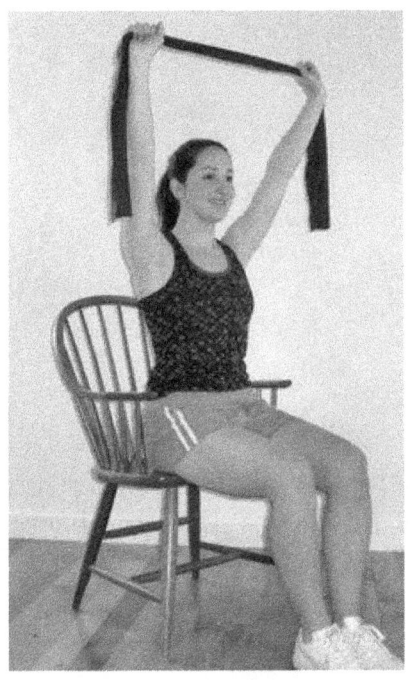

1. Grab a towel and sit tall in a chair with a hard-back.

2. Place your right arm straight down on the chair behind you and hold one end of the towel with your left hand.

3. Lean forward and with your left hand, make a figure 8 over your head and down your left side.

4. Do 8 to 10 reps, and then switch sides.

Abdominal Hold

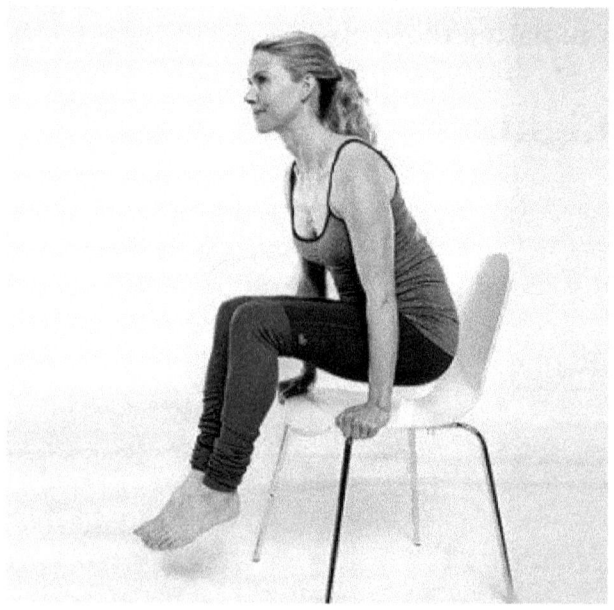

1. Now sit tall on the edge of the chair with your hands on the edge of the seat and your fingers pointing to your knees.

2. Tighten your abs and bring your toes 2 to 4 inches off the floor and lift your body off of the chair. Hold for as long as you can, shoot for 5 to 10 seconds.

3. Lower yourself down and repeat. Continue this exercise for 1 minute. Beginners can keep one foot on the ground for additional support.

Navel Pull-In

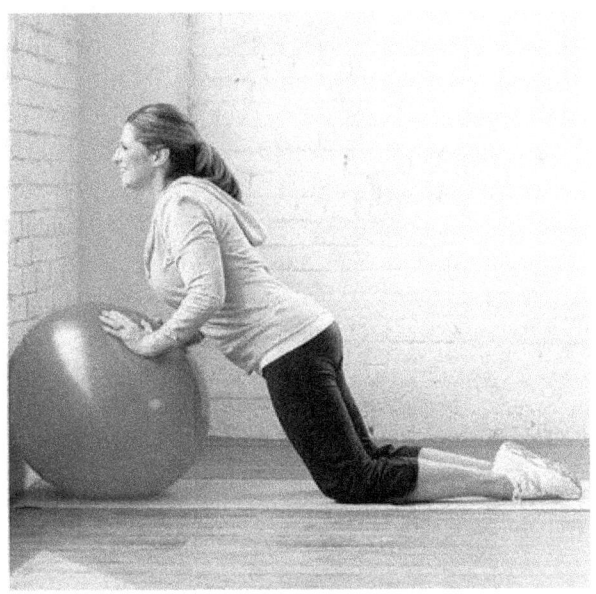

1. Kneel on the floor in front of a chair with your knees hip-width apart.

2. Bend forward at your waist and place your elbows on the chair.

3. Breathe in and exhale, slowly contracting your navel in toward your spine. Pull your navel in and hold for 5 to 10 seconds.

4. Do as many reps as you can each time, building up to 10 reps.

Superman Raises

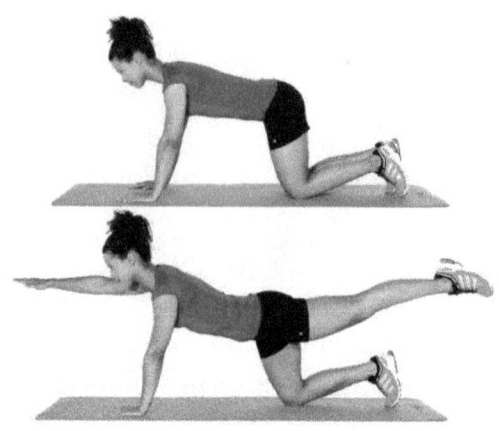

1. Get on all fours, aligning your knees under your hips and hands under your shoulders.

2. Lift your right arm to shoulder height and your left leg to hip height, hold for two counts. Reach forward with your fingers and back with your heel.

3. Repeat this exercise on the opposite side. Do 20 reps, alternating sides.

4. To burn a few more calories, touch your opposite elbow to your knee as you pull your arm and leg in.

Leg Lifts

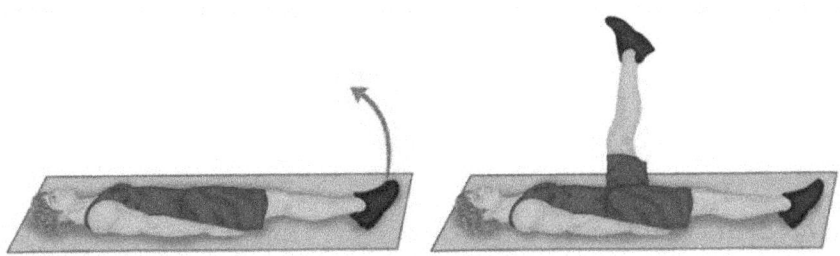

1. Sit up with your back straight on the floor, with your legs stretched out and your toes pointing towards the ceiling.

2. Slowly raise each leg as high as you can, pulling in your abdominal muscles, then lower it. Raise and lower the alternate leg. Repeat the set of raises 20 times.

3. Rest for 20 seconds... then repeat all of the exercises until the 17 minutes is up.

Next Steps

Don't forget, you will not do these exercises again for two days, because you will be working on your legs and butt, so put plenty of energy into it.

There are also a few little tips you can use to help perfect your abs faster and more effectively, so read on...

5 Secrets to Flatter Abs!

The exercise that you will do, both cardio and toning, will take care of giving you a much better body. The food will certain help you shed the pounds. But what about those little tips that go beyond diet and exercise?

Here are few extra secrets for flatter abs:

1. **Don't eat late at night** – This doesn't just mean takeaway pizza, don't eat any meals, however healthy, after 8pm.

    This is because the body will find the late-night calories much harder to burn off and is more likely to hold onto the excess energy in the form of fat.

    Guess where?

    That's right, all around your waist.

    Don't risk more belly fat, only eat before 8pm and try to drink just water and herbal tea after this time too.

2. **Keep on drinking lots of water** – Most people suffer from dehydration on a daily basis, but have no idea why they feel sluggish and find the excess weight hard to shift.

    Remember, we are 60% water. We need to keep ourselves constantly topped up in order to be able to enjoy peak health and lose maximum weight.

3. **Don't skip your snack** – Always eat a light healthy snack in the afternoon. There is a great reason for this and it revolves around insulin.

   A healthy snack boosts your metabolism and balances out your blood sugar. When you keep your blood sugar lower you keep your insulin levels lower.

   Insulin needs to be kept low, because it is what tells your body to store fat around your waist. If you eat every 3 or 4 hours, you avoid the great peaks and troughs in your blood sugar levels, which are detrimental to your health.

4. **Chew well** – Digestion begins long before you swallow. Chew your food properly, until it is ground into a paste in your mouth.

   That way all the right enzymes can work on the food and start to break it down. If you do not chew your food properly, you are likely to suffer from indigestion and bloating, which work against you when you are trying to lose weight.

5. **Laugh a lot!** – This is the most fun tip ever. The diet really will take care of the food side of shifting the weight for you, but this is one of the enjoyable little lifestyle changes that can really help.

   Laughing – deep, spontaneous 'belly laughs' - are just that; they work your belly muscles.

You don't have to spend all day rolling around laughing at jokes (as if you had the time). However, being happy will actually help you to lose weight and studies have shown that feeling down causes people to eat more and exercise less effectively – so keep on laughing!

That's your abs sorted, if you just stick to the plan. Now it is time to take a look at your butt...

Chapter 6

Firm Up Your Butt

Generally moving around more and doing your cardio every morning should seriously help to help tighten you up in this area. However, these exercises are number one when it comes to toning and firming.

Remember, you only do them for 17 minutes at a time. The following evening, you will do the leg exercises in the next chapter, then back to your abs after that and then these exercises again, three days later. This constant rotation will keep you in ever-improving shape.

Here's the fast route to a better butt:

Single Glute Leg Lift

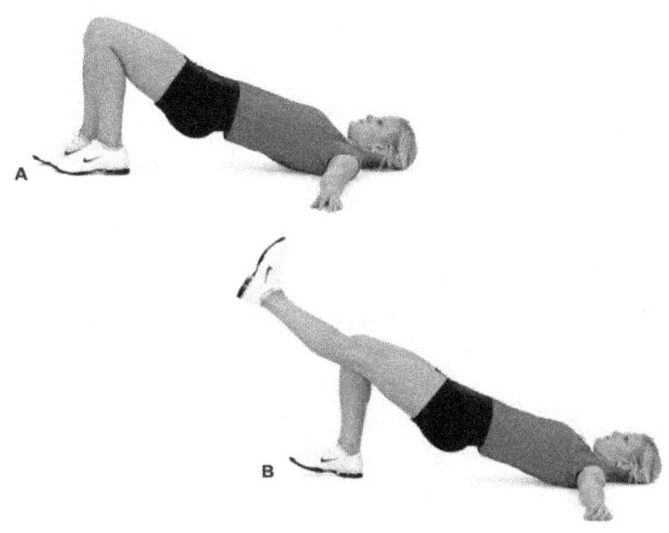

1. Lie on your back with your knees bent and your feet flat on the floor. Extend one leg, squeeze your glutes hard and pushing your hips up toward the ceiling as high as possible.

2. Pause, then lower your leg nearly to the floor (but not touching it), and then repeat x10.

Doggy Kicks

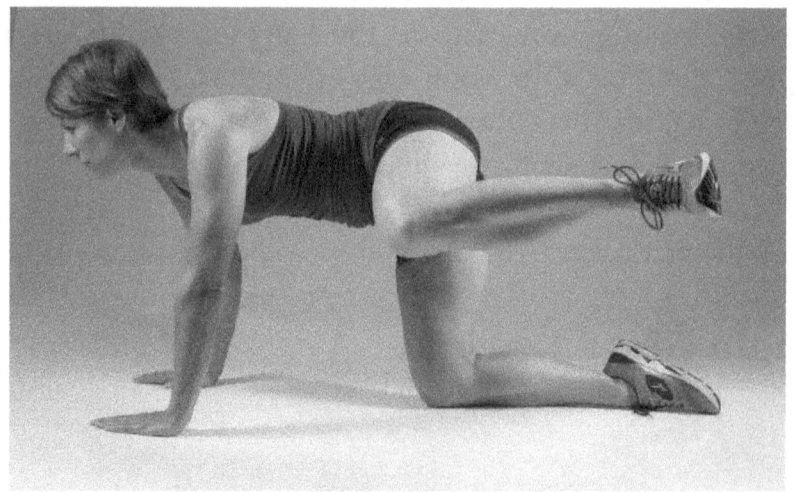

1. Kneel on all fours with your knees hip-width apart.

2. Lift your left knee back toward the ceiling, then extend the left foot straight out to the side. Wait a moment and then bend your knee again, and bring your leg back to starting position.

3. Repeat for one minute on the left side, and then switch to the right.

Curtsy Kicks

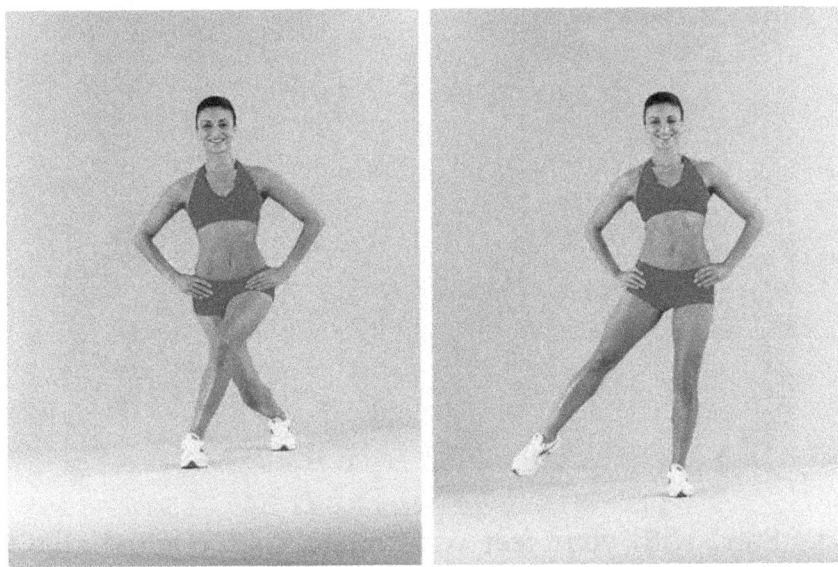

1. Stand with your feet shoulder-width apart and your hands on your hips.

2. Do a shallow curtsy, crossing your right leg behind you and stepping backward in a small dip.

3. Pause, and then extend your right leg into a side kick. Repeat for 1 full minute before you switch legs.

Sumo Tippy Toes

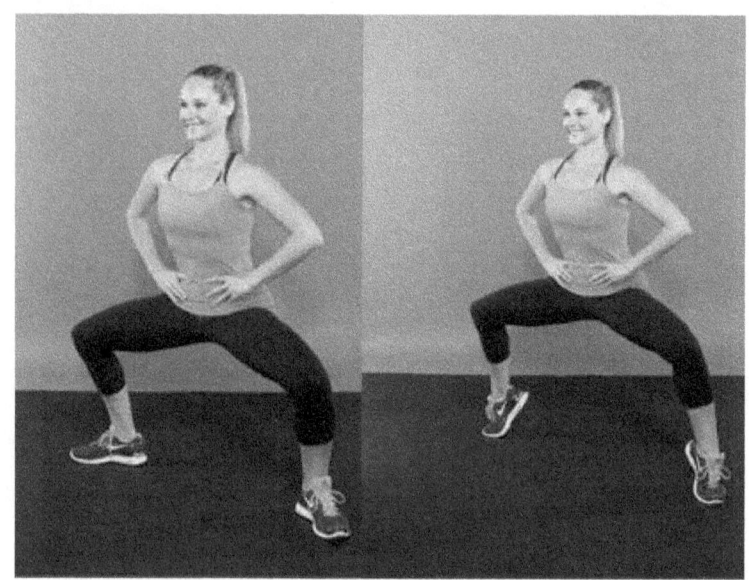

1. Start with your feet wide apart, toes pointed slightly outward, keeping your knees above your ankles and abs drawn in tight.

2. Push your knees back as far as you can and lower your hips toward the floor until your thighs are parallel with the ground.

3. Raise both heels off the ground in a slow and controlled way.

4. Pause, then slowly lower your heels. Repeat 10 times.

5. Now stand and stretch your arms up high, then slowly touch your toes and hold the stretch.

6. Now repeat the whole butt routine 2 more times, or until the 17 minutes is up.

Treat Your Behind

Stay enthusiastic and reward your butt for its improved shape by taking good care of it.

Here are a few top-tips to ensure your butt is well-loved and primed to tighten and shrink:

Try Dry Brushing

Use a special soft bristle bath brush or natural loofah to brush the skin over your bottom.

This will not only exfoliate, ridding your of dead skin cells, it will also stimulate your circulation, which will help rid your body toxins, stored in fat.

Do some dry brushing every day and you will notice a difference, particularly in terms of softer, smoother skin.

It's a Wrap

A natural detoxifying wrap treatment can literally take inches off your behind and help to both break down cellulite and shift toxins.

A treatment that is available at most spas, it involves being covered in the treatment lotion or gel and wrapped tightly to let it penetrate the skin.

This would make a great treat to enjoy when you have completed all 17 days of your slim down – it's a truly relaxing, indulgent and healthy reward.

Once again, thank you for reading this book, and I hope you're getting a lot of valuable information. I would greatly appreciate it if you could take 30 seconds to leave me a review for this book on Amazon.com.

Chapter 7

Want Lean Legs?

Now for some great exercises to get those legs into fantastic shape.

So many of us dislike our legs. We think they are too short, or too heavy, or showing signs of cellulite...

But have you ever thought that rather than hate them, you actually just under-use them?

Legs are amazing, carrying us about everywhere and normally only tiring after the most strenuous activity.

We need to look after them.

Legs love to work hard – the more we give them to do, they are able to do.

The 17-Day Slim Down will help you to rediscover your wonderful legs and they will thank you by slimming down and improving their shape.

Remember, on top of your daily cardio you only do the following leg exercises for 17 minutes, every three days. You simply rotate, working down the body – abs, butt, legs, abs, butt, legs and so on for 17 days.

The leg exercises here are straightforward but highly effective. The trick is to do them as thoroughly as you can... and enjoy!

Leg Lift

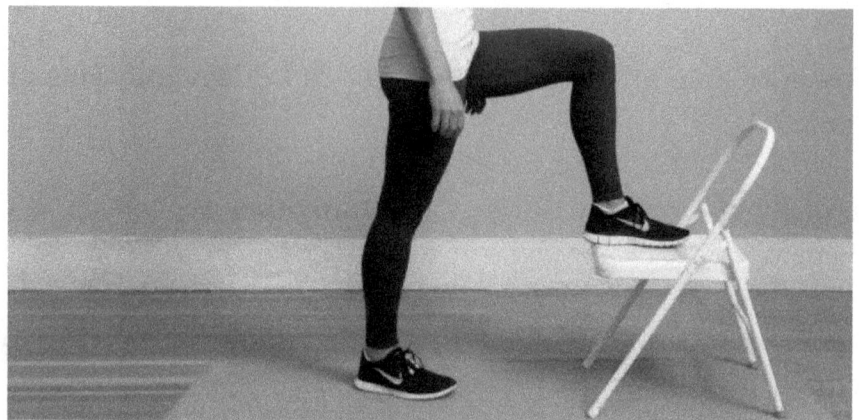

1. Stand facing a chair and raise your right leg, knee facing up, foot flexed and place your heel on the seat. Do not lock your standing knee.

2. Lift your right foot off the chair and straighten it out until you feel your quadriceps working hard.

3. Keep your lifted leg in the air, then bend the leg on the floor slightly and straighten it again.

4. Repeat 15 times then switch sides and repeat for 1 full set. Do 3 sets.

Jump Squat

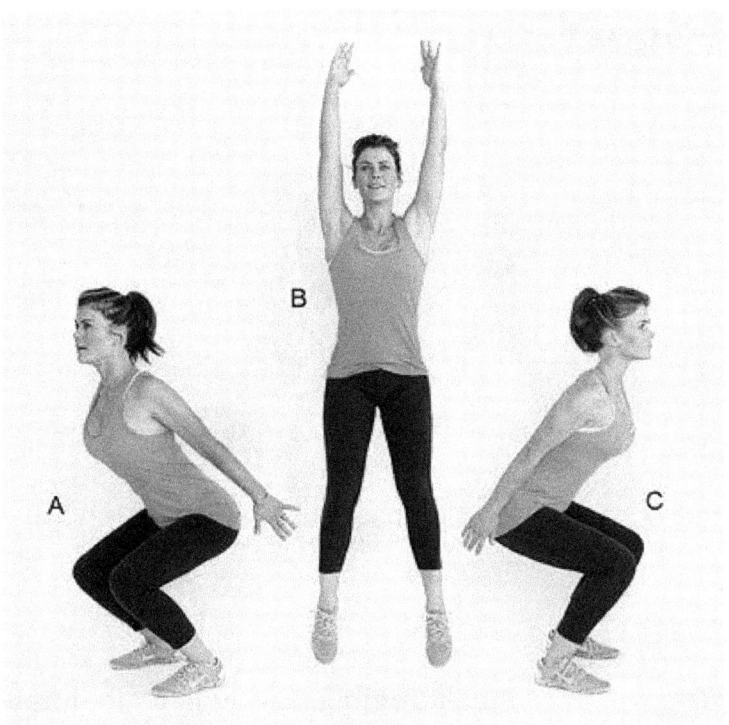

This move is great for quads and hamstrings.

1. Stand with feet shoulder-width apart and arms at your sides. Lower the body into a squat, going two-thirds of the way down.

2. Immediately jump straight up with your arms pointed up toward the ceiling.

3. As soon as you land, start over with the next rep.

4. Do 20 reps to make one set then rest for 15 seconds. Do 3 sets in total

Split-Squat

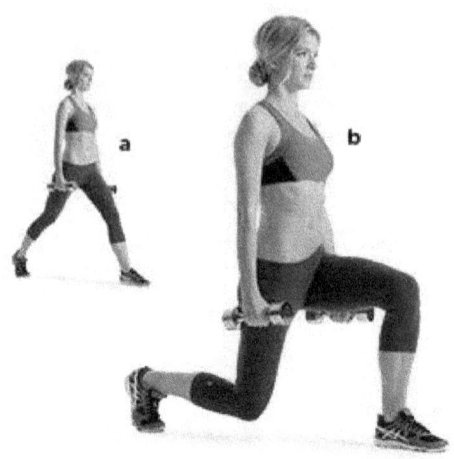

1. You will need small dumbbells – hold a 5lb dumbbell in each hand and keep your arms at your sides.

2. Stand with your left foot far forward and right foot far back. Bend both knees keeping the left knee over your ankle; lower the right knee nearly to the floor. Return to standing.

3. Do 8 reps on each side.

Side-Lift and Kick

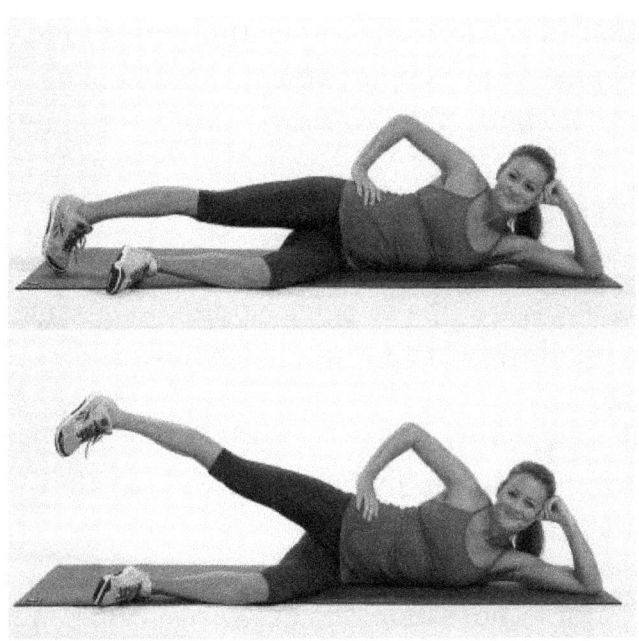

This is a harder move, but worth it.

1. Lie on your right side, leaning your weigh onto your right elbow and tricep.

2. Bend your knees and lift the top bent leg, keeping it level, and then lower it. Straighten both legs and let one leg fall lower than the other.

3. Lower the bottom leg to about 1-2 inches from the floor with knees facing forward. Return to starting position to complete one rep.

4. Do 30 reps, and then switch sides.

5. Do all of these exercises to the max to enjoy the full benefits. When you have completed them all, take a rest for 30 seconds, then start over until 17 minutes are up.

5 Top Tips for Leaner Legs

Here are a few extra tips to get your gets in slimmer shape – keep them in mind even after the 17 days are up.

1. **Take the stairs -** We have evolved from being able to hunt animals for miles or to walk to find sources of water.

   Elevators and escalators obviously came much, much later!

   For fitter, leaner legs, always take the stairs when you can. You'll be amazed at how quickly your body gets used to it.

2. **Leave the car at home** - It is not always possible, but when you have the option of driving and parking, or strolling to your destination, take the latter option. It will take longer, but the health benefits are worth it.

3. **Walk faster** - When you are trying to get from A to B, even if it is just walking across a supermarket car park, try to pick up the pace.

   This will work your legs harder and more often, which ultimately leads to slimmer legs.

4. **Use a standing desk** - A modern solution to the problem that millions of us who are stuck at a desk all day face.

   Essentially, this higher-level desk is designed to be used while standing, which keeps you more active, toned and burning more calories as well.

5. **Get some fresh air** - Don't feel tied to your desk all day (even if it's a standing one).

   Rediscover your local park and go for a brisk, 30-minute, leg-stretching walk every day before you eat your healthy Slim Down lunch. You won't believe the extra energy you feel and your body will think it's Christmas.

Chapter 8

The VITAL Ingredient to Weight Loss

Now we come to the most VITAL factor in your weight loss. VITAL as in Vitamins, Interesting ingredients, Tasty, Amino acid-packed, Life-giving goodness…

That's right – the all-important food!

The 17-Day Slim Down is an easy-to-follow guide to a slimmer, happier, healthier you, which you can achieve by following a simple, nutritious and satisfying diet, based on sound, proven principles.

Many people worry that going on a slimming program will leave them hungry and feeling cranky.

More than that, we have a deep-rooted fear of hunger – it's a primitive response to a lack of food and completely essential for our survival as species. Any successful diet therefore needs not to trigger our survival instincts by underfeeding us.

The 17-Day Slim Down provides all the nutrition you need to feel great and lose weight, without the hunger pangs.

The food plan offers plenty of choice and a real variety of healthy foods. Here's the lowdown on the main principles of the diet.

Your 17-Day Food Plan

This remarkably effective weight-loss plan is based on eating mainly whole, fresh foods. That means no processed foods, no high-salt foods, or food with added sugars. It is a weight-loss plan that is designed to work with your system, not against it. This means avoid any foods that will aggravate your digestion or cause adverse reactions.

For example, to minimize the risk of bloating, the 17-Day Slim Down largely excludes foods that typically form gas, which means no beans, cabbage, onions, peppers, cauliflower, brussel sprouts or dried fruit.

Some people also experience a bloating reaction when they eat apples, watermelon and chewing gum containing sorbitol, so avoid these at your discretion if this applies to you.

Throughout the 17-day period, you also need avoid all alcohol and caffeine, so don't drink regular coffee or tea (herbal infusions and rooibos are fine) and make sure that you avoid all energy drinks. This might sound like quite a few things to avoid. The reality, though, is that you will have a great deal of freedom when it comes to choosing your meals during the 17-Day Slim Down.

Remember, as discussed earlier, you can select the meals you want from our wide selection for breakfast, lunch and dinner, plus you can enjoy a daily snack. You can eat the snack whenever you like, or even add it to one of your three meals if you prefer.

This much you already know. But you are in for a nice surprise when you see the food on offer. The meals in this plan are not designed to starve you skinny. That would only backfire badly when, being totally ravenous, you start to each again and your body immediately stores fat.

We have not evolved to waste away, our metabolic survival mechanisms can unfortunately work against us so that our bodies hold tightly onto every last calorie...

This slimming plan is different. It is low in fat, high in fiber, both soluble and insoluble.

The insoluble fiber aspect is extremely important because this fiber is not digested in the stomach and small intestine, so it passes on into the colon, sweeping through it like a natural brush. Insoluble fiber soaks up water to form a soft bulky mass, which moves easily along the digestive tract.

Having a high-fiber diet, like this one which recommends whole foods, aids your digestion and also helps you to fill fuller for longer and for fewer calories, all of which greatly helps with weight loss.

By only recommending whole foods healthy amounts and cutting out the empty calories in sugary, fatty or processed foods, not only will you not starve, but also you will receive all the best nutrients and plenty of fiber.

Your digestion will function properly and your metabolic rate, aided by the exercise you are doing, will increase. Ultimately, your body will respond favorably by dropping the pounds.

The Water Factor

Drink a lot of water throughout the 17-Day Slim Down. Begin your day with a refreshing, rehydrating, cleansing glass of water and lemon, end the day with water, perhaps in the form of an herbal tea like chamomile and drink plenty of water all day long.

Water has countless benefits for the body.

First, it keeps you fully hydrated, which is essential for your body to function properly. It also flushes out toxins more effectively, plus it keeps your metabolism and digestion all fired up, which is the best news for anyone who is trying to lose weight.

Water fills you up so you are less tempted to snack, it quenches your thirst and best of all it contains zero calories. Make it your best friend through the whole of the next 17 days and beyond. Try to drink 6-8 large glasses each day.

So now, back to the food. What is the best way to approach mealtimes during your 17-Day Slim Down so that it remains totally effective and enjoyable?

Planning Your Meals

This is a really easy and enjoyable part of the diet. You can browse through the all the various delicious recipes and meal ideas, simply selecting one breakfast, lunch, dinner and snack per day.

As there are plenty to choose from – 17 in each section - you can tailor the eating plan to your own tastes. If you have wide-ranging tastes, simply have a different breakfast, lunch, dinner and snack every day, or have the same few several times over – it's your call.

In any case, if you stick to the plan you will get the right nutritional balance to lose weight and a nice variety of foods to enjoy.

To make planning your meals even easier, we have provided a full Shopping List, which contains everything you can possibly need for ALL the meals.

Buy it all and make every single meal over the course 17 days, or pick and choose depending on the particular meals you have selected – again, your call.

We have not specified strict amounts as that will depend on the choices you make and we do not want you to over-buy unnecessarily.

To make things easier still, at times in the meal plan, we will specify that you need to eat 1 portion of fruit. We do not dictate which fruit this must be as everyone has their own particular favorites.

Instead, we also provide some Fruit Portions, which lists some suggestions as to which fruits you might like to snack on, along with the recommended portion size.

This is not an exhaustive list, but it can be helpful when you want to know, for example, how many grapes you would be advised to eat as your fruit portion.

To keep things really simple, of course all of these fruits are also included in the main shopping list, for ease of reference.

One additional point about your shopping. Do try to go for the best quality fresh ingredients that you can afford. This does not necessarily have to mean the most expensive, although if you choose to go organic this normally comes with a higher price tag.

If you can afford go organic, do. There has been some debate about whether eating organic produce is any different to eating regular fruit and vegetables. In truth, most of the time it really is different.

Organic fruit and vegetables have been grown without the farmer using any chemicals - no artificial fertilizers or pesticides – and in accordance with very strict guidelines.

This results in virtually unadulterated organic fruit and veg which has been proven to be much higher in antioxidants and much lower in its levels of toxins, metals and pesticides.

In a brief summary of some of the findings of the Organic Trade Association, they have found that growing organically really does make a measurable difference to the composition of the produce when compared to conventionally grown fruit and vegetables.

In a famous study, the significantly higher levels antioxidants in organic crops included:

- 19% higher levels of phenolic acids
- 69% higher levels of flavanones
- 28% higher levels of stilbenes
- 26% higher levels of flavones
- 50% higher levels of flavonols
- 51% higher levels of anthocyanins

These antioxidants have been shown to lower the risk of heart disease, brain diseases and certain cancers.

If you switch to eating only organic fruit and vegetables, you will enjoy a 20-40% increase in the antioxidants you consume, without upping your calorie intake.

This phenomenal antioxidant pay-off (in addition to on average 48% less of carcinogenic metal cadmium) is a pretty good reason to consider going organic when you set off with the Shopping List in Chapter 15!

Fruit Portions

As outlined earlier in the book, this list gives you a selection of roughly equivalent fruit portions, for when '1 portion fruit' is specified in your meal plan. Choose your favorites, but try to keep your choices varied if possible.

- 1 apple
- 4 apricots
- 1 banana

- 1 cup mixed berries
- 1 cup blueberries
- 2 figs
- 1½ cups fresh fruit salad
- ½ grapefruit
- 12 grapes
- 1 guava
- 1 kiwi fruit
- ½ mango
- 1 cup melon
- 1 orange
- 4 passion fruit
- 1 cup pawpaw
- 1 peach
- 1 pear
- 4 rings pineapple
- 2 plums
- 3 prunes
- 2 satsumas
- 1½ cups strawberries
- 1 slice watermelon

Enjoying this book?

Check out my other best sellers!

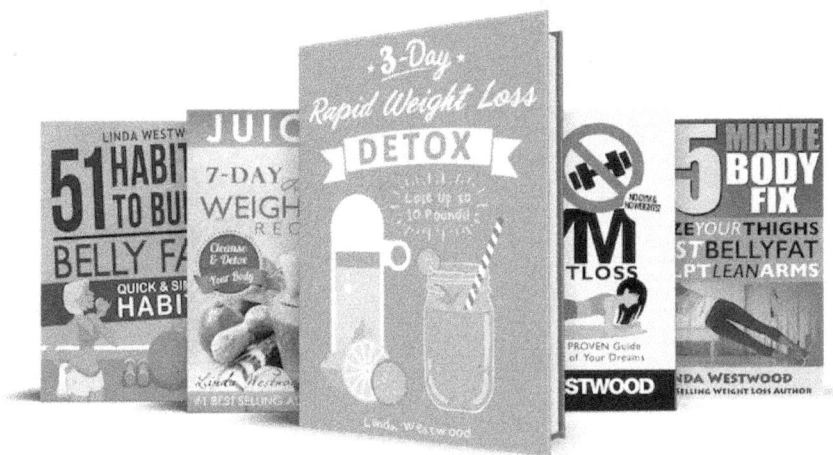

Get your next book on sale here:

TopFitnessAdvice.com/go/books

Chapter 9

Breakfast Options

Breakfast is the meal that gets our metabolism fired up for the day. We are literally breaking our fast that came with a good night's sleep and our body's systems are requiring the right fuel.

A good breakfast is therefore absolutely essential if you want to enjoy a healthy start to the day.

We have therefore recommended some delicious, well-balanced and highly nutritious recipes and breakfast ideas, which will fill you up, rev up your metabolism and ultimately help you lose weight.

Above all other meals, you need to have a decent breakfast, so don't ever be tempted to skip it. Many respected studies have shown direct links between people who are overweight and people skipping breakfast.

Conversely, those who are trying to lose weight are more likely to succeed when they eat a good, healthy breakfast.

Moreover, when it comes to exercise, you need to fuel your inner fires to be able to perform properly – after all, you will be carrying out daily 17 minutes of cardio plus your legs, butt and abs workouts each day and regular breakfast eaters exercise more effectively.

Finally, when you eat a proper breakfast you tend to eat fewer calories overall during the day. You are basically less likely to 'cheat' on your slim down because you will already be feeling satisfied.

Also, when you browse many of the breakfasts, you'll notice that we recommend that you also enjoy one piece of fruit as part of your meal. This gives you an early boost of nutrients and fiber each and every day – plus it will taste wonderful!

So, don't hold back!

Go ahead and pick out some great breakfast recipes to look forward to during your 17-Day Slim Down. They are likely to be one of the main keys to your weight-loss success.

Bran Slam

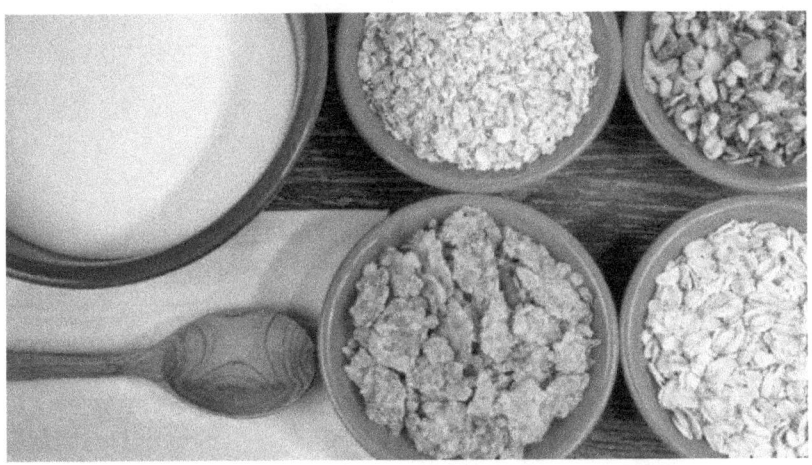

Fill up nicely by enjoying some healthy bran flakes for breakfast. Bran is a superb food – it is basically the hard outer layer of cereals and it is incredibly high in fiber, as well as essential fatty acids and other nutrients.

Eating bran for breakfast, along with the fruit, will help you feel full and help keep your digestive system working smoothly.

Ingredients

- 1 cup organic bran flakes
- 2/3 cup fat-free milk
- PLUS 1 portion fruit – Try sliced banana on top of your bran flakes, delicious.

Egg and Tomato Burrito

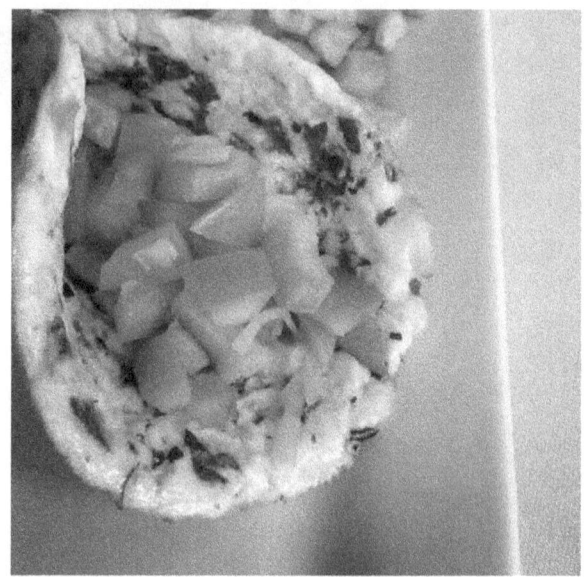

Eggs have, on occasion, had a bad press, but in truth they do not raise bad cholesterol in most people. They are low calorie and they are protein-packed and super-nutritious, making them one of the true secret weapons of the dieter.

Nutrients include Vitamins A, B2, B5, B12, B6, D, E and K, plus folate, selenium, calcium and zinc – amazing!

This healthy burrito recipe, makes the most of your eggs, topped off with tasty low-fat cheese and fresh, super-healthy tomato for a great start to your day.

Ingredients

- 2 eggs
- 1 tbsp low-fat milk

- 1 tbsp low-fat cheddar cheese
- 1 fat-free whole-wheat tortilla
- 2 tomatoes
- A few sprigs of cilantro
- Low-calorie cooking spray
- Salt and pepper to taste
- PLUS 1 portion fruit

Method

1. Whisk the eggs and milk in a medium bowl. Season lightly.

2. Coarsely chop the tomatoes.

3. Spray the low-fat cooking mist onto a nonstick skillet with cooking spray over low heat. Add the egg mixture, and stir with a spatula to scramble.

4. Sprinkle the cheese down the center of the tortilla top with the scrambled egg, 2 tablespoons tomato and sprinkle with torn cilantro.

5. Roll up in the style of a burrito, i.e. by folding the bottom up and bringing the sides into the center. Eat immediately.

Oat So Easy

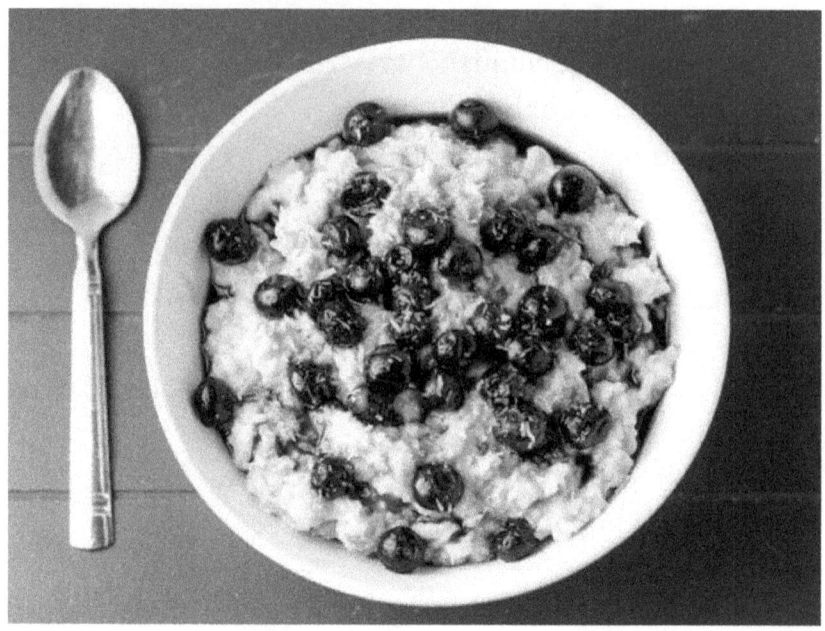

Oats are essential for heart health and can even help to combat diabetes. They contain a special fiber, which can be incredibly effective at lowering cholesterol levels.

Moreover, they fill you up and they taste great!

Ingredients

- ½ cup unsweetened oats
- 2/3 cup fat-free milk
- PLUS 1 portion fruit. If you fancy making your oats nice and fruity, try stirring in some blueberries.

Method

1. Heat the oats and milk in a saucepan, occasionally stirring. Alternatively, place the oats in a microwaveable bowl, pour over the milk and heat on high for 2 minutes.

2. Remove and stir, then heat again on high for a further minute, or until the oats have a creamy appearance.

Breakfast Margherita

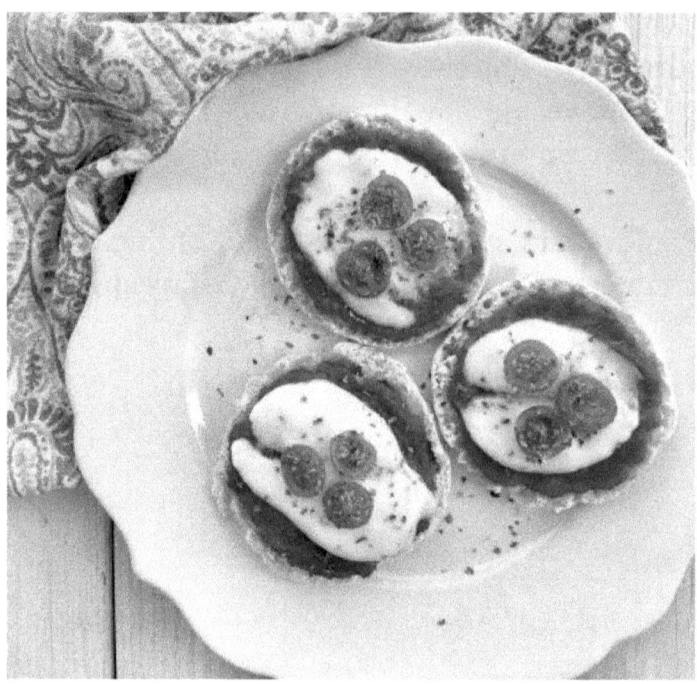

With the dough of the bread topped with cheese, tomato and a scattering of basil, this morning treat reminds us of the world's most popular pizza.

Happily, this version has none of the excess calories and fat – in fact the reduced-fat cottage cheese will just give you a great burst of protein, Vitamin B12, riboflavin and other nutrients - so tuck in!

Ingredients

- 2 slices whole-wheat (seed or rye bread)
- 2 tomatoes (sliced)

- 3 tbsp low-fat cottage cheese,
- A few leaves of fresh basil (dried will do if not)
- PLUS 1 portion fruit

Method

1. Toast the bread. Top it with sliced tomatoes and the cottage cheese, then finish with a scattering of basil. Delicious.

Grilled Cheese and Egg Toasty

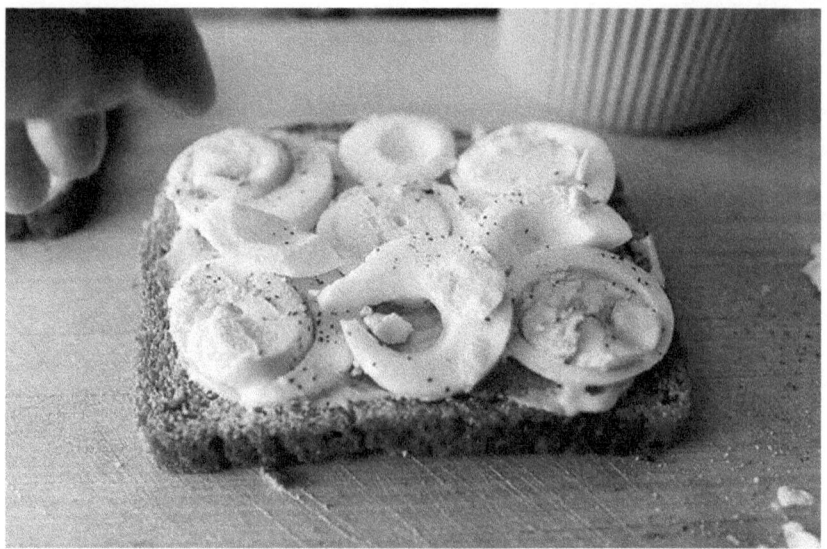

Cheese is often seen as the dieters' enemy, but the low-fat versions that are available in the supermarkets now can be absolutely wonderful for a reduced calorie calcium hit.

This breakfast feels indulgent, but is the perfect choice to twin with a light, leafy lunch to ensure a really varied nutritional balance.

Ingredients

- 2 slices whole-wheat/seed bread
- 30g low-fat cheddar cheese
- 1 boiled egg
- PLUS 1 portion fruit

Method

1. Lightly toast the bread, then top with cheese and place under the grill, meanwhile boil your egg. If you like it hard-boiled, you can slice it up and lay on the cheesy toast, or eat it separately soft-boiled if you prefer.

2. To make a more substantial savory open toasty, you might like to a replace your fruit portion with some slices of ripe tomato instead – technically, it counts as a fruit!

Breakfast Berry Smoothie

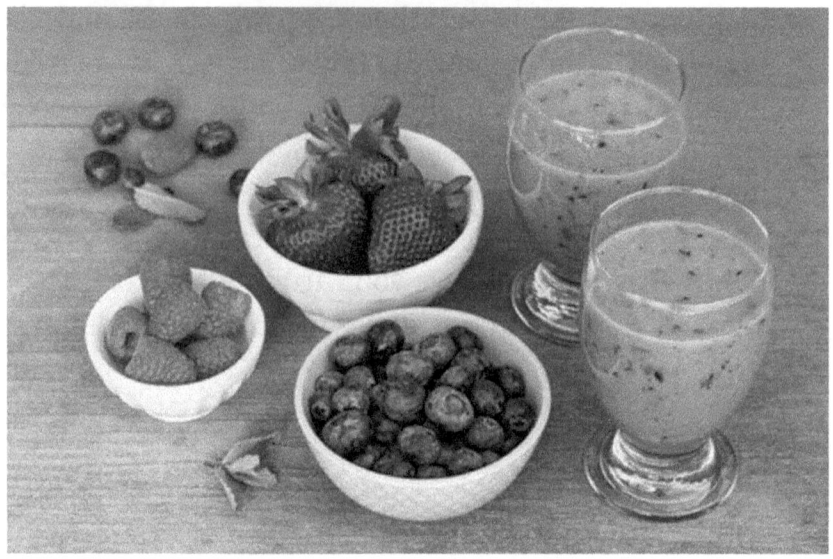

The beauty of this delicious breakfast smoothie is that it is full of vitamins, minerals, protein and fiber – the wheat germ is great for the immune system and helps to prevent all kinds of diseases, at the same time as being great for weight loss.

Meanwhile this smoothie is low in fat but as tasty as any milkshake. Perfect for a guilt-free indulgence early on in the day.

Ingredients

- 1 1/4 cups fresh berries
- 3/4 cup fat-free plain yogurt
- 1/2 cup orange juice
- 2 tablespoons nonfat dry milk
- 1 tablespoon toasted wheat germ

- 1 tablespoon honey
- 1/2 teaspoon vanilla extract

Method

1. Put all the ingredients into a blender and whizz up into your gorgeous smoothie.

Note – your portion of fruit is already included in your breakfast, in the form of the berries, so you don't need extra.

Quick Apple Quinoa

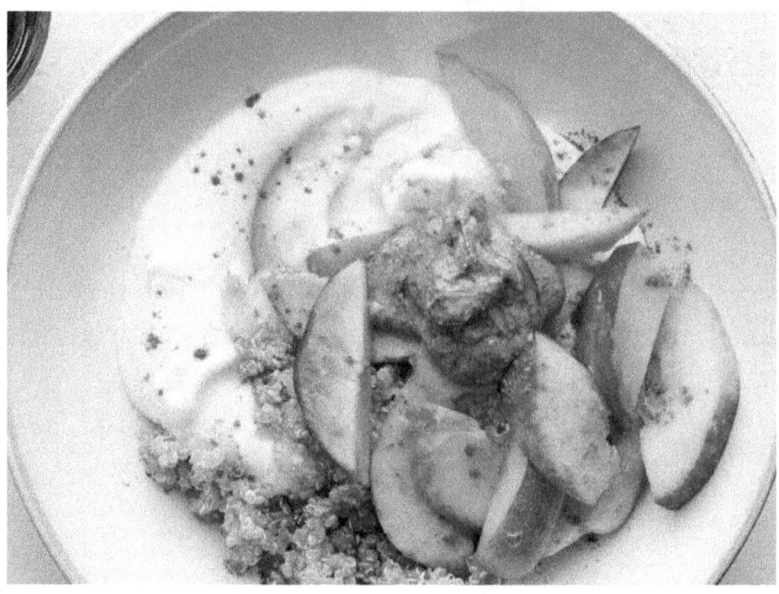

Quinoa has become more of a regular staple in the cupboards of healthy homes in recent years, but many people still have not tried this high-protein grain. Often it is used who to replace rice or Couscous at lunch or dinner, but quinoa flakes make a fabulous alternative to oats or the usual cereals.

Quinoa is a totally tasty superfood, containing all nine essential amino acids and making it a fantastic source of protein.

Ingredients

- 1 cup water
- 2/3 cup quinoa flakes
- 1 tsp cinnamon (+ more for sprinkling)

- 2 tsps vanilla extract
- 1/2 cup unsweetened applesauce
- 1 apples (chopped)

Method

1. Bring water to a boil. Take it off the heat and stir in the quinoa flakes, cinnamon, and vanilla extract. Cover with a lid and let it rest for 1 minute.

2. Stir in the applesauce. Pour the mixture into a bowl and sprinkle it with the chopped fresh apple and sprinkle a touch more cinnamon on top.

Broccoli Feta Omelet

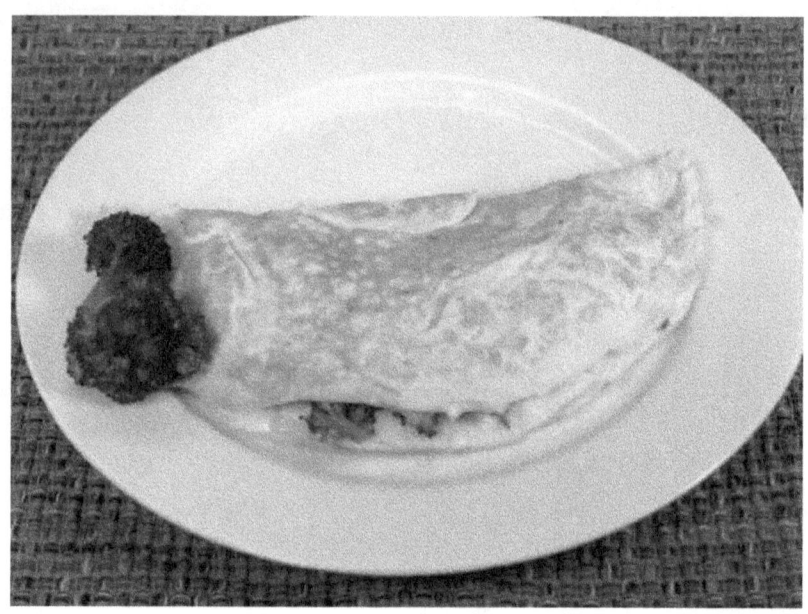

Broccoli is one of the best and most popular superfoods. Certain tests have proven broccoli to be active in preventing the development of, or shrinking, cancer tumors which is pretty amazing for this tasty green veg.

More importantly for your 17-Day Slim Down, it is ultra-low in calories, but full of fibre and nutrients. Feta is already one of the lower calorie cheeses, but buy a good quality reduced fat version

Ingredients

- 1 cup chopped broccoli
- 2 large eggs (whisked)
- 1 tablespoon reduced-fat Feta cheese (crumbled)

- 1/4 teaspoon dried dill
- Low-cal cooking spray
- 1 slice rye bread (toasted)

Method

1. Gently heat a nonstick skillet over medium heat and with the low-cal cooking spray. Add the broccoli, and cook for 3 minutes.

2. Mix the eggs, Feta and dill in a bowl, whisk and then pour into the pan.

3. Cook for 3-4 minutes then fold the omelet in half with a spatula and cook for 2 more minutes or until ready. Serve with the rye toast.

Florentine Bake

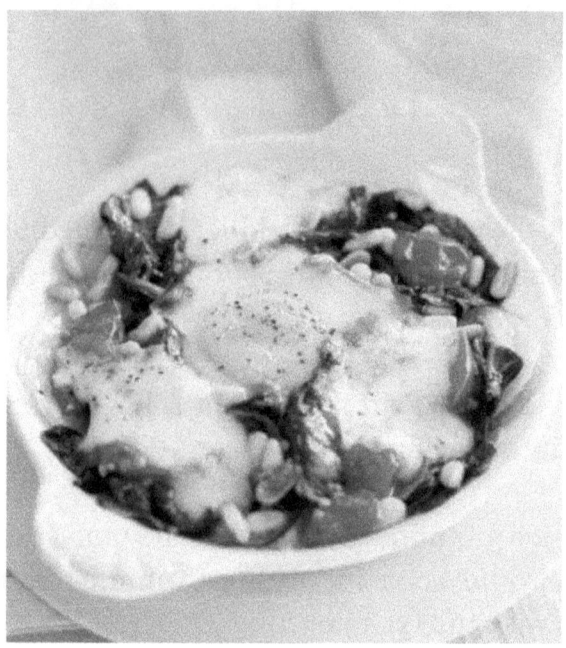

Eggs and spinach make a great, very healthy combination. We already know that eggs provide a shellful of low-calorie, super-nutritious goodness.

But spinach is an amazing food too – cleansing the blood and a powerful source of both iron (remember Popeye?) and Vitamin C. All these nutritional goodies will give your body a great boost and support you as you shed the pounds – great news as you enjoy this very tasty and satisfying dish.

Ingredients

- A handful of bag spinach
- 1 tbsp chopped tomatoes

- 1 tiny pinch chili flakes
- 1 egg

Method

1. Heat oven to 200C/180C fan/gas 6. Place the spinach into a small size and pour over a little boiling water from a kettle to wilt it.

2. Press the spinach with a fork to squeeze out the excess water and place into 1 small ovenproof dish.

3. Mix the tomatoes with the chili flakes and season, then add to the dish as well.

4. Create a small well in the center of the dish and crack in the egg.

5. Bake for 12-15 mins or more depending on how you like your eggs.

Cranberry Raspberry Smoothie

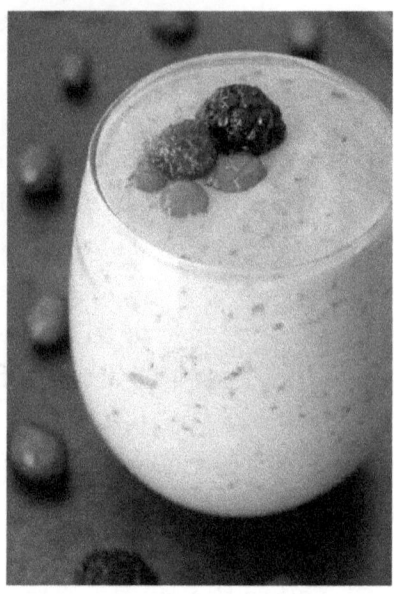

Super low-calorie cranberries are great for your health and deliver a nice sweet-sour flavor to perk up the taste buds of anyone who is losing weight. They boost immunity, help to keep your blood press excellent for warding off urinary tract infections, plus they boost immunity, lower blood pressure and taste great.

Ingredients

- 200ml cranberry juice
- 175g frozen raspberries (defrosted)
- 100ml milk
- 200ml natural yogurt
- Mint sprigs (to serve)

Method

1. Place all the ingredients into a blender and pulse until smooth. Pour into glasses and serve topped with fresh mint.

Sunny Green Soldiers

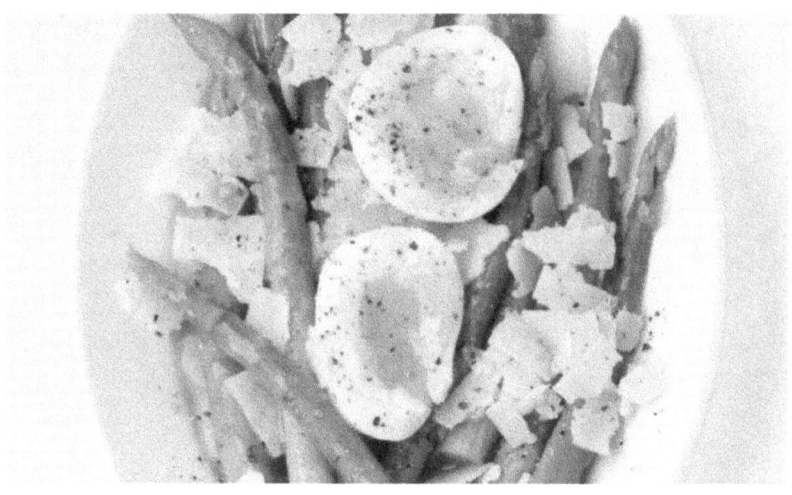

Enjoy a simply but totally healthy light breakfast when you prepare a soft-boiled egg with asparagus spears instead of soldiers. The egg will set you up for the day with a blast of nutrients and protein.

Meanwhile, asparagus, with its refined and delicious taste, is a natural diuretic and contains high levels of vitamin K, plus folate, vitamin B12, selenium, vitamin B2, vitamin C, vitamin E and much more.

Moreover, each average size spear only contains 3 calories, which is amazingly low for all the goodness and flavor you will gain. So eat up in confidence that you are still doing wonders for your waistline.

Ingredients

- 5 asparagus spears

- 1 egg
- PLUS 1 portion fruit

Method

1. Cook the asparagus in a large pan of boiling salted water for 3-5 mins until tender.

2. At the same time, boil the egg for 3 mins.

3. Put the egg in an egg cup on a plate, drain the asparagus and serve alongside it. Just dip and eat, no spoon required!

Creamy Fruit Bowl

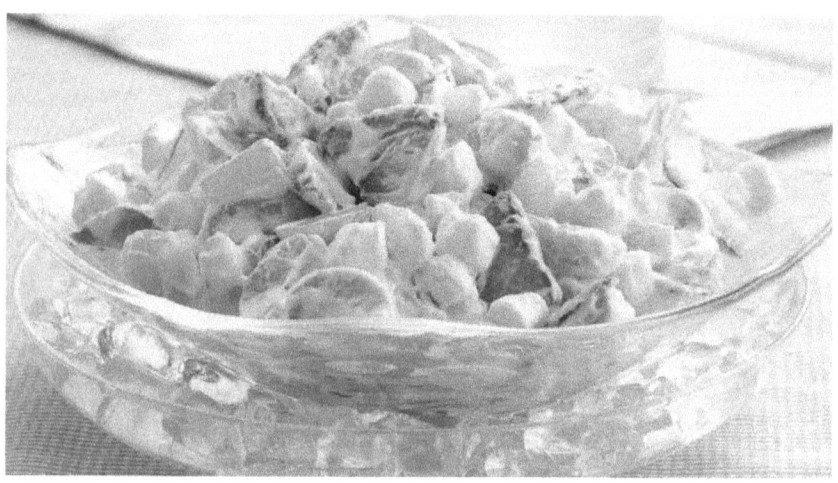

Something, nothing more is needed that a simple bowl of fruit, made all the more creamy and delicious but adding that tasty and super low-cal alternative to cream, fat-free natural yoghurt. The fruit itself provides a heady, body-loving cocktail of every vitamin under the sun and plenty of fiber. Meanwhile, the fat-free natural yoghurt offers some exceptional benefits.

As well as the calcium that is essential for bone health, a celebrated study showed that dieters who ate some yoghurt daily lost more belly fat and retained more lean muscle than those in the same study who did not eat yoghurt. Food for thought.

Ingredients

- 1 cup fresh fruit salad
- 2 tbsp fat-free natural yoghurt

Whole-Wheat Salmon and Eggs Deluxe

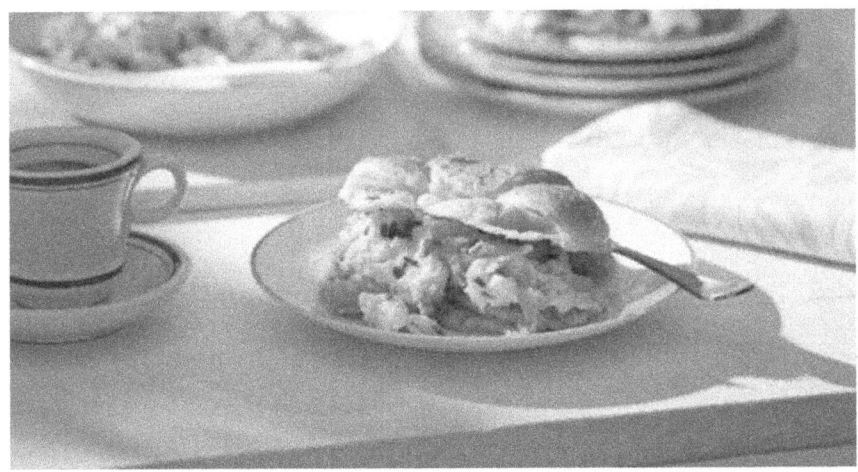

Where to start with the health benefits of this delicious breakfast? The eggs and salmon will give you a perfect protein hit, which your body will thank you for.

The super-nutrient combination in eggs is topped up by the B vitamins, vitamin D, magnesium, selenium, DHA, EPA and omega-3 fatty acids in the tasty salmon.

The whole-wheat muffin will fill you up with fiber and helps to make this into a great meal. Eat this when you want lots of slow-burning energy for a demanding day.

Ingredients

- 2 large eggs
- 1 thin slice smoked salmon (diced)
- Few leaves of chopped fresh spinach

- 1 splash of fat-free milk
- 2 tsp reduced-fat cream cheese
- 1 whole wheat English muffins (split and toasted)
- Low-cal cooking spray
- 1 tsp chopped chives
- 1 pinch freshly ground black pepper
- PLUS 1 portion fruit

Method

1. Mist some of the cooking spray into a medium nonstick skillet and turn it onto a medium heat.

2. Whisk the eggs, milk and pepper a bowl until well combined.

3. Pour egg mixture into skillet and cook until the mixture begins to thicken, continuously stirring it with wooden spoon.

4. Stir in the salmon and cream cheese and cook for 30 seconds, breaking up any lumps of cream cheese with a spoon.

5. Stir in the spinach for cook 2 more minutes or until spinach wilts and the eggs are just cooked, stirring constantly.

6. Top each muffin half with 1/2 of the egg mixture and garnish with the chives.

Waffle with Blueberries

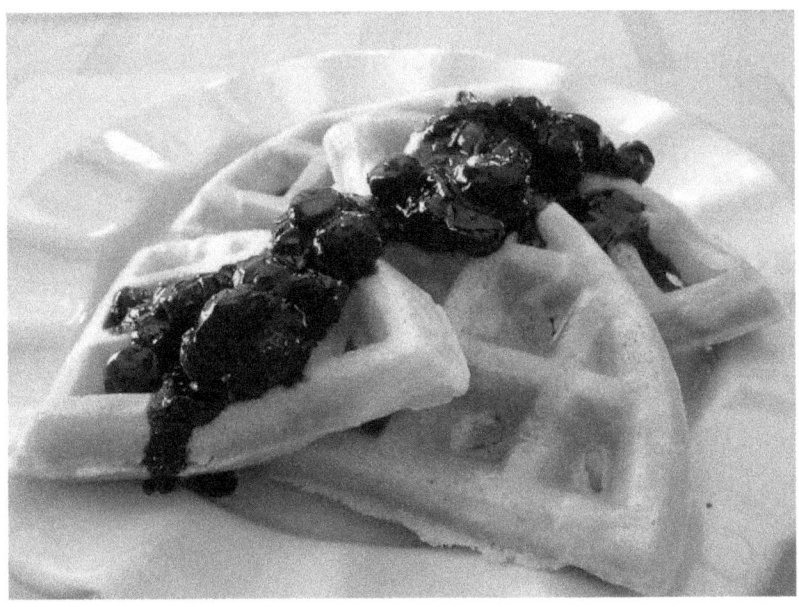

This 17-Day Slim Down focuses on helping you to get slim with the best possible foods, with a whole foods as a focus. Waffles may seem like an indulgence, but we don't mean the over-processed type that are full of added sugar.

Look out for the artisan-made, organic, whole-wheat type of waffle, or if you own a waffle iron and are feeling adventurous, then go ahead and make your own.

Ingredients

Quick recipe for one

- 1/3 cup frozen blueberries
- 1 teaspoon maple syrup

- 1 whole-grain waffle
- 3 or 4 pecans
- If you have a waffle iron, it is even better and more wholesome to make your own…

Makes 4-5 waffles (serve one waffle per person)

- 2 large eggs
- 1 ¾ cups fat-free milk
- 1 tbsp light olive oil
- 1 tbsp honey
- ½ tsp ground cinnamon
- ¼ teaspoon baking soda
- 1 ½ cups whole-wheat flour
- 2 teaspoons baking powder
- 1 tiny pinch of salt

Method

To make waffles

1. Preheat your waffle iron.

2. Whisk the eggs, milk, oil, honey, cinnamon and baking soda together in a mixing bowl until well combined.

3. Add in the whole-wheat flour, baking powder, and salt and whisk together until the mixture is completely smooth.

4. When the waffle iron is hot, drizzle over a little olive oil and then ladle some batter onto the center of the iron.

5. Cook according to the instructions for your waffle maker, normally about 3 or 4 minutes.

6. Store each waffle on a warm plate in the oven until they are all ready.

To serve

1. If you are serving several people, increase the amount of berries, syrup and pecans accordingly.

2. Microwave blueberries and syrup together for 2 to 3 minutes,
   until berries are thawed.

3. Top the toasted waffles with warm blueberries and sprinkle with pecans.

Poached Egg Tricolore

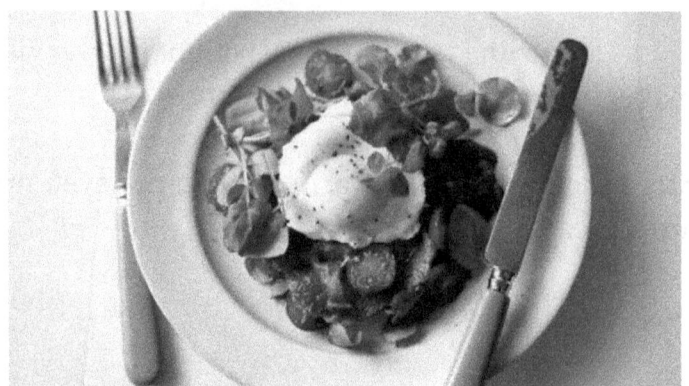

We already know that eggs and tomatoes are delicious, nutritious, colorful additions to any meal. But sit them on a large bed of peppery, dark green watercress and they are transformed into a fresh yet rich and satisfying brunch-style meal.

Watercress is yet another one of nature's gifts to dieters. It is full to the brim with Vitamin K (among other top nutrients), which helps with healing the body and strengthening bones. This is a really tasty savory breakfast treat.

Ingredients

- 1 egg
- A handful watercress
- 1 tomato
- Salt and pepper to taste
- Drop of vinegar
- PLUS – 1 portion fruit

Method

1. Poach your egg according to your favorite method – some people user egg-poachers, others do it the old-fashioned way. If you've never poached an egg before, this is a foolproof technique.

2. Put on a medium-sized saucepan of water to boil and add a pinch of salt to it.

3. Make sure your egg is really fresh and crack one into a ramekin or cup. Add a small drop of vinegar to your egg.

4. When the water is boiling, take a hand-held balloon whisk and stir the water to create a gentle whirlpool in the water, which will help the egg white wrap around the yolk.

5. Slowly tip the egg into the water, white first. Turn the heat right down to the minimum setting. Leave to cook for three minutes.

6. Remove with a slotted spoon, snipping off any straggly edges using the edge of the spoon.

7. Rest the egg to drain onto kitchen paper – this is an important step as a waterlogged dish is unpleasant.

8. Serve the egg on a large bed of watercress and wedges of tomato.

Blueberry Oat Sundae

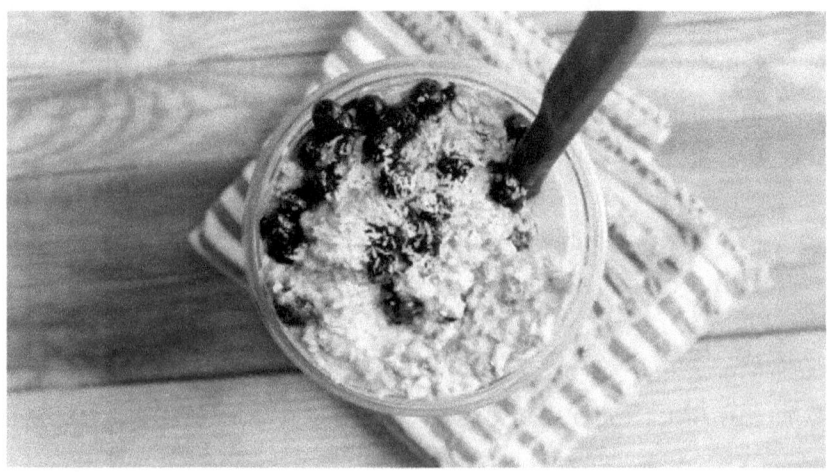

Blueberries are dark little flavor bombs that are simply exploding with nutrients. They are a good source of vitamin K and also contain vitamin C, fiber, manganese and other antioxidants.

The great news for dieters is that they are very low in calories, yet they are totally tasty sweet treats. This recipe looks and tastes great and you could even use it as a dessert if you have guests to dinner during your 17-Day Slim Down.

Ingredients

- 25g (1oz) oats
- 3 tbsp fat-free Greek yogurt
- ½ tbsp honey
- 50g (2oz) blueberries

Method

1. First toast the oats by tossing and stirring them around in a dry frying pan for 1 or 2 mins until golden.

2. Mix together the yogurt and honey and place half in a sundae or wine glass.

3. Then sprinkle half the toasted oats into the glass. Top with half the blueberries then repeat the layers.

Note - This oat and yogurt layered treat is even more delicious after it has been chilled in the fridge for at least an hour beforehand.

Forest Omelet

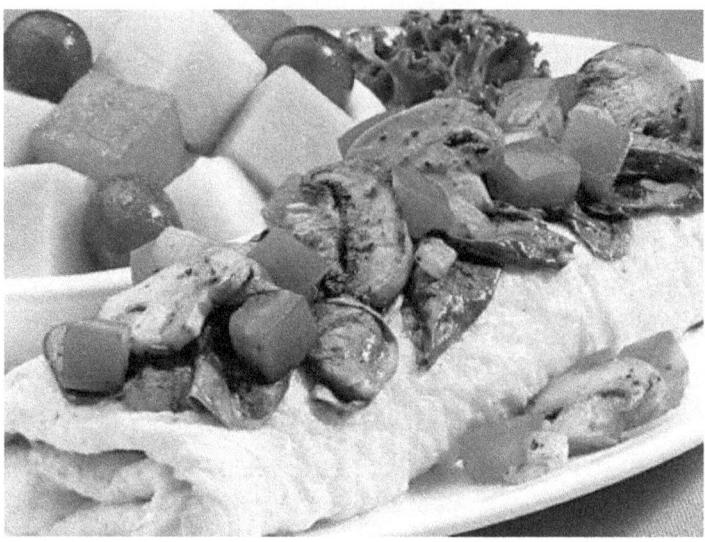

This is a delicious, filling breakfast to enjoy, where the stars are mushrooms, asparagus and eggs, all earthy and very wholesome ingredients.

The trick with all three is to obtain them super-fresh so they are at their very best in terms of taste and nutritional value and, critically, not to overcook them.

Mushrooms have very few calories and have the added benefit of having been shown in studies to enhance weight loss.

Ingredients

- 1/4 cup chopped, fresh asparagus
- 1/4 cup sliced mushrooms
- 1 large egg

- 3 large egg whites
- 1 tbsp fat-free milk
- 1 small pinch of salt
- A dash of black pepper
- 1/4 cup reduced-fat mozzarella cheese (1/2 ounce)

Method

1. Put a small, non-stick skillet onto a medium-high to heat and mist with low-calorie cooking spray until it is evenly coated.

2. Fry the asparagus and mushrooms for four minutes, or until tender. Remove them and set aside on a warm plate.

3. Whisk the egg, egg whites, milk, salt and pepper together in a small bowl.

4. Pour the egg mixture into the pan, coating the entire bottom of the pan and allow to cook for 2 minutes.

5. Sprinkle the cheese, mushrooms, and asparagus on one half of the omelet.

6. Use a spatula to fold one end of the omelet over the other, so that all the vegetables are enveloped inside.

7. Continue cooking for 2 more minutes, until egg is fully cooked through. Slide the omelet onto a plate and eat immediately.

If you're enjoying this book and would love to let other potential readers know how great it is, please take a few seconds to leave a review on Amazon.com.

Chapter 10

Lunch Options

Now onto the next exciting recipe selection – your choice of lunches. These lunches are all very varied, so there will definitely be something here for all tastes.

These lunches give you energy and boost your mood while filling you with vital nutrients, all for relatively few calories – in weight-loss terms that is the same as hitting the jackpot!

In this chapter, the recipes offer plenty of lean protein in the delicious form of salmon, tuna, chicken, and even a little lean beef to keep things interesting.

Every recipe has some leafy or vegetable bulk to it to, so that it taste fresh and delivers on the fiber. Plus, many have healthier forms of carbohydrate, like soba noodles or wheat berries to give you the wholesome, wholegrain goodness.

A great lunch can make all the difference to your day. If you are someone who usually grabs the nearest processed, greasy, packaged offering that you can find to swallow in five minutes at your desk, you will soon notice a major difference in how you feel during the afternoon after you have had a truly healthy and enjoyable lunch.

We know that not everyone has the time to cook intricate dishes in the middle of their busy day. We have therefore kept things largely very simple and many of the dishes can be made in advance and stored for whenever you need them, or taken to work in a lunchbox.

The key thing to remember is that as these lunch dishes are mostly high in fiber, so you may even feel that you are eating more food than usual.

For example, a large bowl of chicken and vegetable soup will fill you up as least as much as a cheese and ham sandwich and a packet of potato chips, but it has a fraction of the fat and under a quarter of the calories.

Fiber is the filling dieter's friend. It is great for the digestive system and it features strongly in this chapter.

This is a very good thing as you will not be tempted to give in by grabbing high-calorie snacks and you will also have plenty of energy to really perform when you exercise each day.

Plus, all of these dishes taste great, so what are you waiting for?

Summery Tuna Wrap

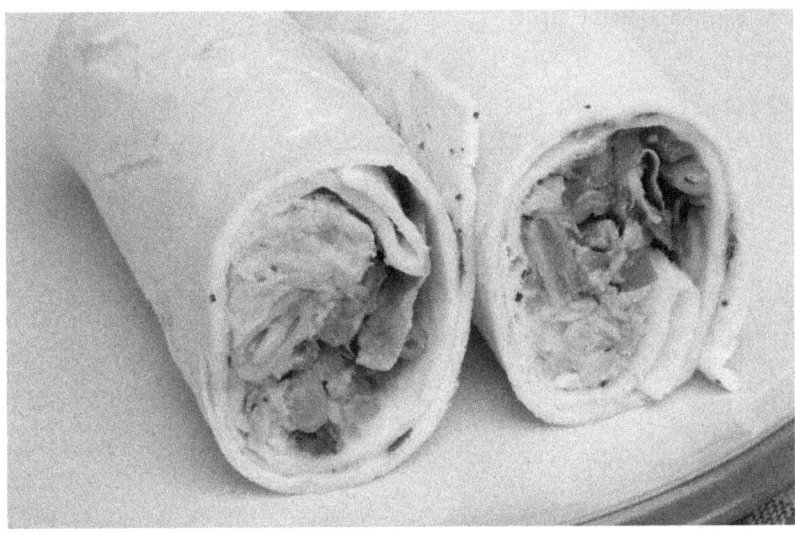

This is a fabulous recipe which uses Greek yogurt to replace the classic, calorific mayo for a low-fat, low cholesterol and creamy alternative.

Tuna is a fantastic ingredient and should be a staple in any store –cupboard. It is very rich in protein and tastes light and savory, plus it will fill you up. Although it is named after the hottest months, thanks to the delicious fresh yogurt and the salad vegetables, it is ideal for lunch at any time of year.

Ingredients

- 1 whole-wheat wrap
- ½ a 6oz can of tuna
- ¼ cup non-fat Greek yogurt
- ½ a celery stalk (chopped)
- 3 cherry tomatoes (halved)

- A handful of baby spinach
- A squeeze of lemon juice
- PLUS 1 portion of fruit

Method

1. Blend the tuna with the yogurt.

2. Layer the vegetables into the wrap, spoon on the tuna and squeeze over some lemon. Done!

Light Mediterranean Turkey Burger

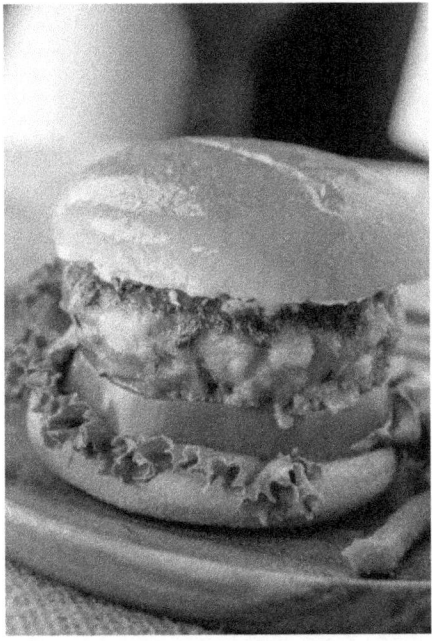

Tasty turkey burgers are super-low in fat and high in protein – they really are a dieter's friend.

You can easily make your own by simply binding freshly seasoned turkey mince with a little beaten egg, shaping them into patties, wrapping the in cling film and freezing them individually until you need to use them.

Ingredients

- 1 whole-wheat bun
- 1 turkey burger patty
- 2 tablespoons reduced-fat feta cheese
- 2 slices tomato

- 1 handful spinach
- Low-calorie cooking spray
- PLUS 1 portion of fruit

Method

1. Coat a skillet in low-calories cooking spray and heat on a medium-high heat.

2. Fry the turkey burger patter for 7-10 minutes or until it is cooked through.

3. Place the patty in the bun and top it with the vegetables and cheese. Good to go!

Super-Veg Sub

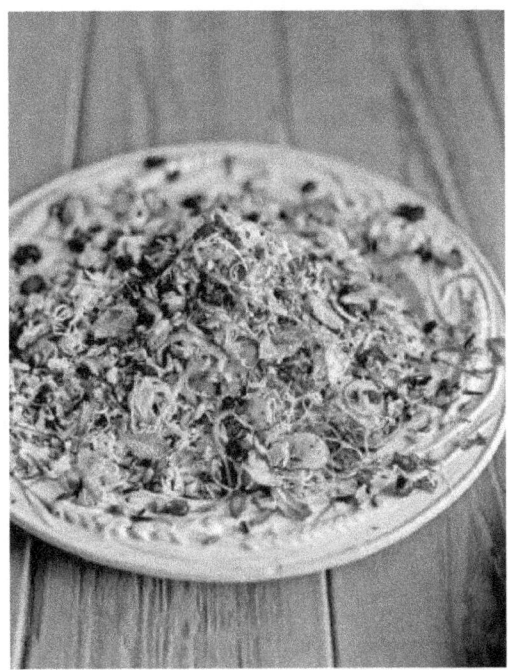

Doctors recommend that you eat 5 portions of fruit or veg per day and this little beauty of a sub contains all 5 and more. It is simply bursting with fiber and vitamins, not to mention all kinds of delicious fresh flavors.

Alfalfa is a sprout which makes a particularly wonderful addition to any meal, seeing at it is packed with nutrients like protein, calcium and other minerals, plus B vitamins, vitamin C, vitamin D, vitamin E, and vitamin K. A true superfood!

Ingredients

- ½ 6-inch whole-wheat sub roll
- 1 tablespoon reduced-fat hummus

- ¼ cucumber (sliced)
- 1 small tomato (sliced)
- 3 black olives (halved)
- ½ carrot (shredded)
- A handful of alfalfa sprouts
- PLUS 1 portion fruit

Method

1. Spread the inside of the half sub with the hummus.

2. Layer on the other colorful veg and top off with the alfalfa. Perfect!

Super-Light Salmon Caesar Wrap

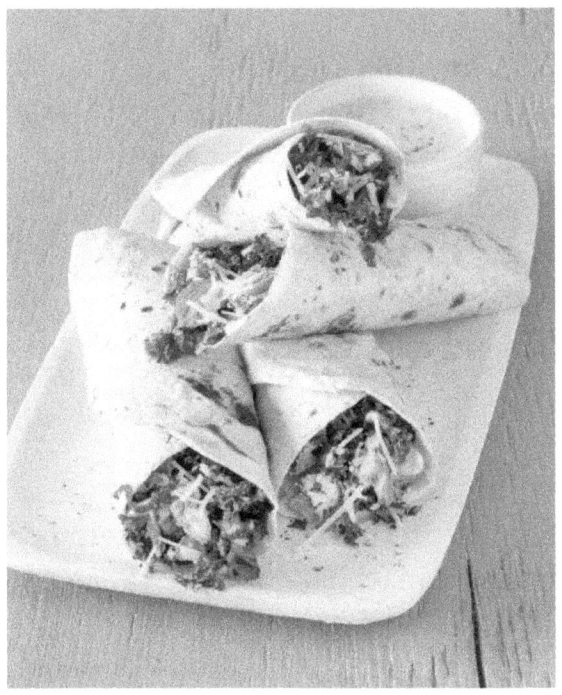

Salmon is amazing for both weight loss and heart health, being full of Omega-3 fatty acids, potassium, selenium, Vitamin B12 and more. The light yogurt dressing is a real winner too.

Ingredients

- 1 whole-wheat pita
- 5oz fillet of salmon, grilled, cooled and flaked (or canned salmon if you are in a hurry)
- 1 handful fresh spinach

For the Dressing (makes enough for at least two wraps)

- ½ cup fat-free Greek yogurt
- 2 tbsp olive oil
- 2 tbsp lemon juice
- 1 clove garlic (pressed)
- 1 pinch each salt and pepper
- ¼ cup grated parmesan cheese
- PLUS 1 portion fruit

Method

1. Cut the pita bread to make a pocket and stuff it with salmon and spinach.

2. Spoon over half the yogurt Caesar dressing, the rest will keep in the fridge for a few days.

Tuna and Arugula Open Sandwiches

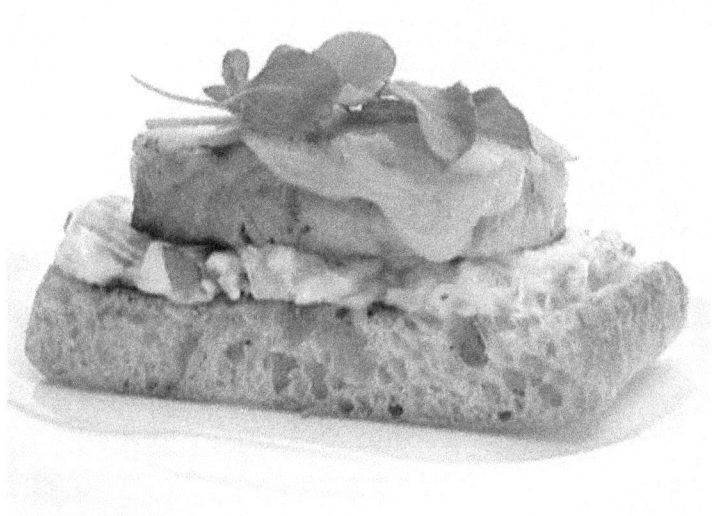

Ingredients

- 2 slices whole-wheat/seed/rye bread
- ½ can tuna in spring water
- 1 heaped tsp homemade fat-free mayo (see recipe below)
- A handful of fresh arugula
- Chopped celery

For the Fat-Free Mayo

- 6 oz. fat-free plain yogurt
- 1/4 tsp cider vinegar
- 1/8 tsp mustard

- 1 dash hot pepper sauce
- 1 pinch of white pepper
- 1 pinch of paprika
- 1 pinch of salt
- PLUS 1 portion fruit

Method

1. Combine all the fat-free mayo ingredients and whip with a fork until creamy.

2. Combine the tuna with the mayo.

3. Layer the arugula onto the bread and top with the creamy tuna, then sprinkle over the chopped celery. Ready to go!

Spring Veg Citrus Salad

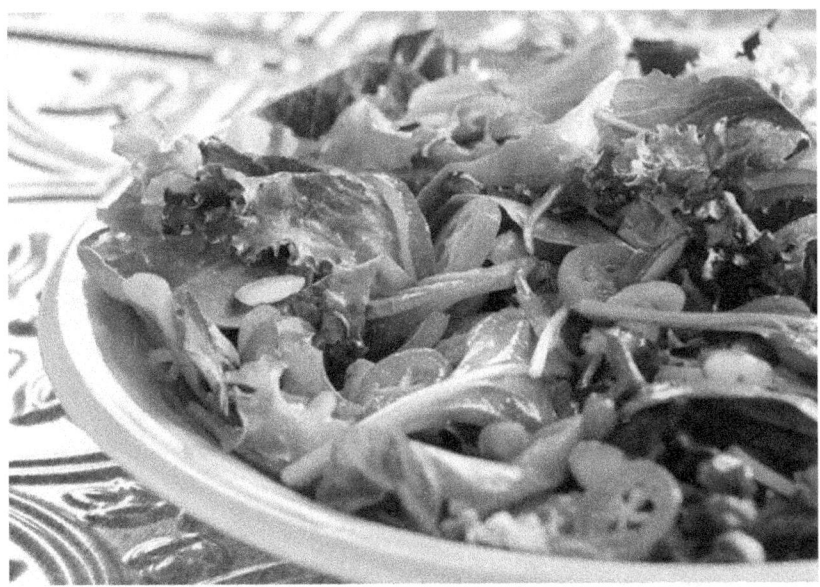

Choose the stunning citrus-accented salad whenever you fancy a real burst of golden sunshine on your plate. Zucchini are a great vegetable.

It is another type of squash and squashes are typically low in calories and high in fiber, plus they even help to prevent certain cancers, so you can never eat too many.

Ingredients

For the Salad

- 1 ½ cups julienne-cut zucchini
- 1 ½ cups julienne-cut yellow squash
- 1 cup fresh corn kernels

- 1 tbsp finely chopped fresh flat-leaf parsley
- 1 tbsp finely chopped fresh basil
- 1 tbsp chopped chives

For the Vinaigrette

- 3 tbsp fresh orange juice
- 1 ½ tbsp fresh lime juice
- 2 ½ tsp extra-virgin olive oil
- 2 tsp honey
- 1 tsp red wine vinegar
- A pinch of salt and freshly ground black pepper

Method

1. Combine all the salad ingredients together.

2. Combine all the vinaigrette ingredients together.

3. Mix the two and – hey presto! A delicious vegetable salad bursting with fresh flavors.

Egg, Tomato and Avocado Sandwich

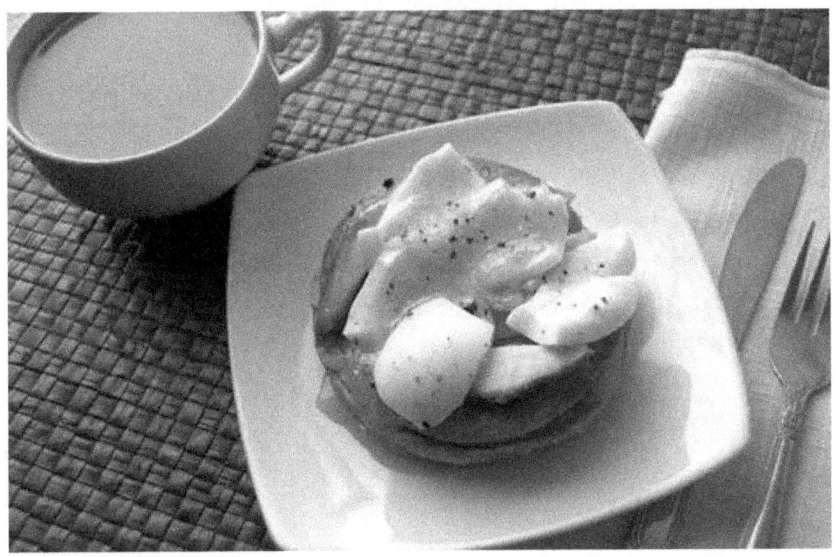

This lean, mean, gorgeously green sandwich is much better for weight loss than your traditional bacon, egg, and cheese muffin.

This light lunch features avocado, a food that nutritionists love. Full of the 'good fats' that we all need, it a rich and highly nutritious component of this super-sandwich. Enjoy!

Ingredients

- 1 whole-wheat English muffin
- 1 large egg (poached)
- ¼ avocado (sliced)
- 2 slices tomato

Method

1. Poach the egg according to the foolproof recipe earlier the book (in the Breakfast Recipes chapter).

2. Layer the avocado and tomato onto the whole-wheat muffin.

3. Place the poached egg on top and enjoy the hot-cold flavor sensation.

Tarragon Chicken Salad

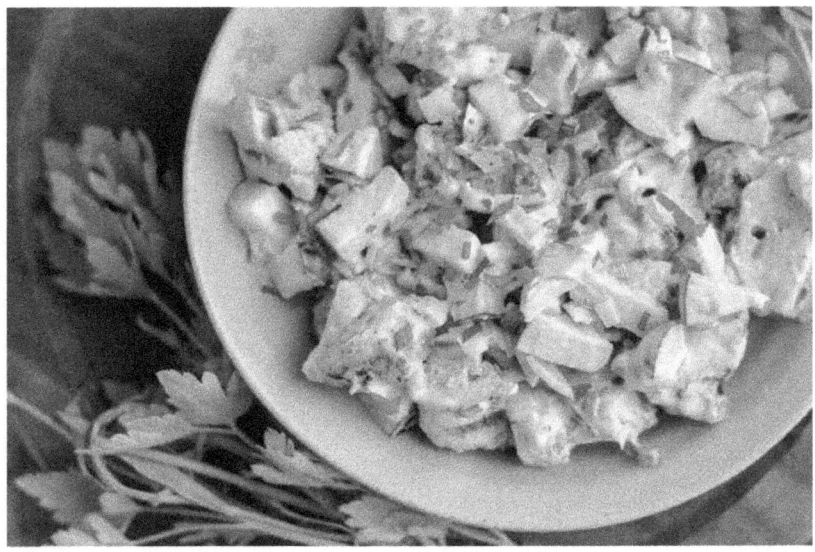

Like avocados, walnuts are also filled with 'good fats' that help the mind and body. Good news for dieters is that they help you feel fuller and have been shown to aid weight loss.

Ingredients

- 1 cup spinach
- ½ a chicken breast (sliced)
- ¼ cup fat-free Greek yogurt
- ¼ cup walnuts
- ¼ cup dried cranberries
- 1 stalk celery (chopped)
- 2 slices tomato
- 1 tablespoon fresh tarragon (chopped)
- 1 squeeze lemon juice

Method

1. Combine all the ingredients and toss them around so that they are fully coated with the Greek yogurt with its squeeze of lemon. Your salad is ready.

Egg Salad Supreme

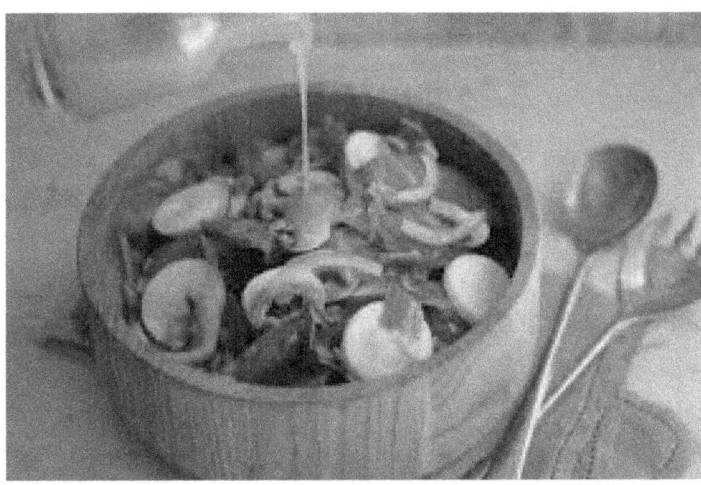

Plenty of protein and fiber in this lovely, healthy lunch, which makes it absolutely ideal for anyone who is trying to lose weight.

The peppery salad, tasty egg and low-fat cheese also ensure that there is no compromise when it comes to flavor.

Ingredients

- 1 hard-boiled egg (cooled)
- 3 tbsp low-fat cottage cheese
- 1 tbsp fresh parsley (chopped)
- A small handful of arugula
- A small handful of watercress
- 1 slice rye bread to serve
- PLUS 1 portion fruit

Method

1. Make a bed of greens from the watercress and arugula. Slice the hard-boiled egg and layer it over the salad.

2. Spoon over the cottage cheese. Sprinkle over the chopped parsley and enjoy with a slice of plain rye bread.

Chicken Bulgur Salad

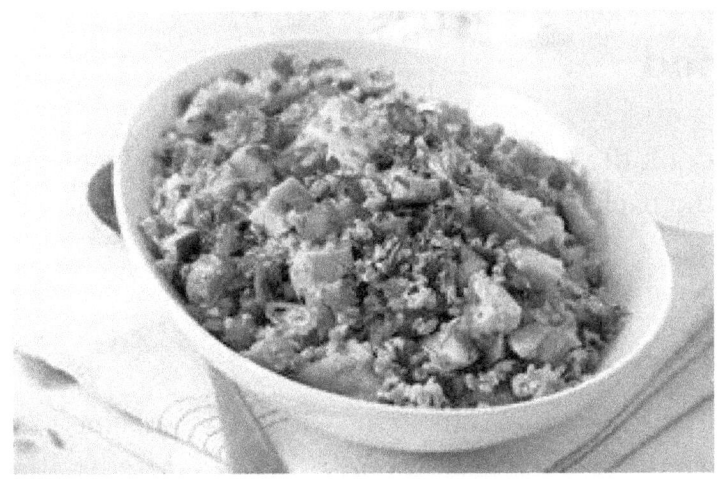

Bulgur wheat has enjoyed greater popularity in recent years and with good reason. It is a great heart-healthy source of fiber, protein, iron and vitamin B6.

Also, as a wholefood, it will keep you filling fuller for longer, a great benefit when you are trying to lose weight.

Ingredients

- 1 cup bulgur wheat
- 1 small chicken breast
- 1 tbsp pumpkin seeds
- 1 tbsp honey
- 1 tbsp white wine vinegar
- ¾ tbsp olive oil
- 2 tsp Dijon mustard
- 6-8 cherry tomatoes (halved)
- ¼ cucumber (diced)

- A handful of fresh cilantro (chopped)
- PLUS 1 portion fruit

Method

1. Cook the bulgur wheat according to the instructions on the packet.

2. Meanwhile, grill the chicken breast until it is cooked through, then cut it into roughly bite-sized pieces.

3. Combine the chicken with the drained bulgur, cucumber, cherry tomato halves, tossing them all together.

4. Place the honey, olive oil, white wine vinegar and mustard in a small bowl and use a fork to whip it into a dressing emulsion.

5. Pour the dressing over the chicken and bulgur wheat, sprinkle over the chopped cilantro and the pumpkin seeds.

Light Greek Salad Wrap

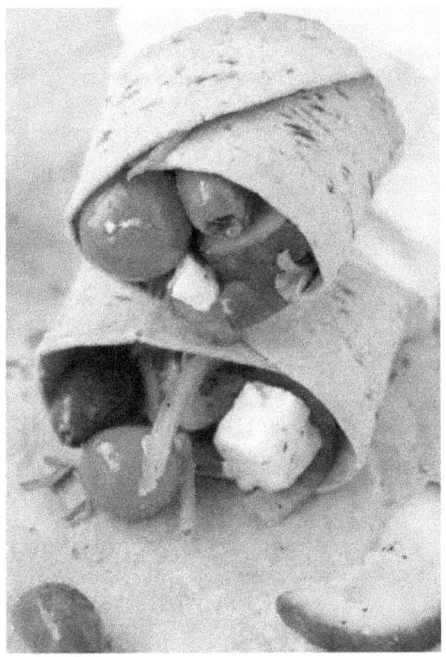

This clever little lunch comprises all the elements of a classic Greek salad – olives, tomatoes and cucumber, but replaced the feta with super-light cottage cheese.

Olives can be a good ingredient on a diet, not just because they contain healthy fats, vitamin E and minerals, but also because their strong, distinctive flavor helps to take the edge of hunger, leaving you feeling satisfied.

Ingredients

- 1 whole-wheat tortilla wrap
- 8-10 pitted olives
- 2 tomatoes (diced)

- ¼ cucumber (diced)
- 3 tbsp low-fat cottage cheese
- A few leaves of fresh basil
- PLUS 1 portion fruit

Method

1. Lie the tortilla flat on the plate and spoon the cottage cheese, cucumber and tomato into the center, sprinkled with the olives and basil.

2. Fold the tortilla by bring the sides into the center and the bringing the bottom edge up to the middle, then enjoy.

Citrus Shrimp Salad

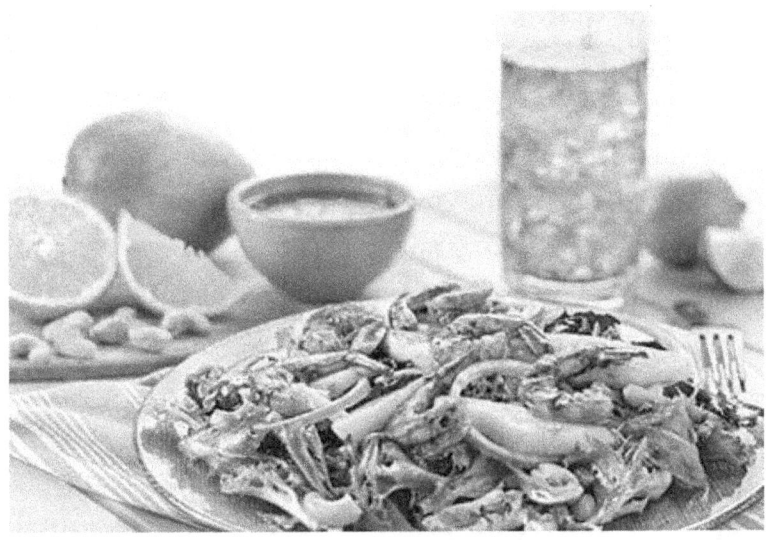

There are few things as delicious as freshly cooked shrimp, especially when you are watching the calorie count. Shrimp are a real seafood treat, plus they are very nutritious.

They are absolutely full of selenium and are a unique source of astaxathin, an antioxidant and anti-inflammatory nutrient. Selenium can help to ensure a strong thyroid function, which is essential for anyone who wishes to control their weight.

Ingredients

- 3oz raw shrimp
- A large handful of mixed lettuce leaves
- ¼ cup chopped fennel
- 1/3 avocado (sliced)
- 1 tbsp lemon juice

- 1 tsp olive oil
- Juice of half an orange (plus segments of the other half)
- Juice of half a pink grapefruit (plus segments of the other half)
- 1 garlic clove
- 2 tsp sunflower seeds
- 2 tsp Parmesan shavings
- Low-calorie cooking spray

Method

1. Sauté the shrimp with the crushed garlic and lemon juice in a skillet coated with the low-calorie cooking spray. Combine the lettuce and the chopped fennel.

2. Whisk together the olive oil and citrus juice, then toss the dressing together with the mixed greens, avocado, shrimp and citrus segments.

3. Top with the Parmesan shavings and sunflower seeds.

Asian Roast Beef Wrap

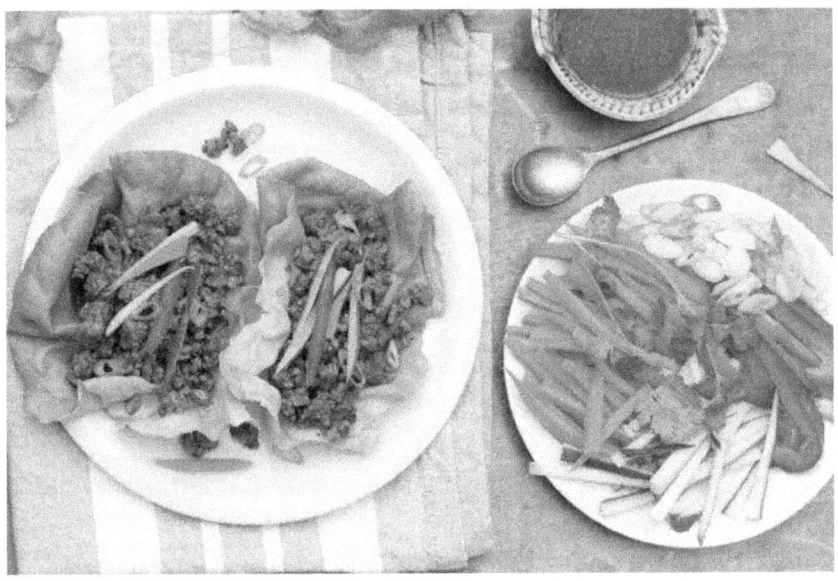

This is a truly delicious and healthy lunch that uses fresh lettuce to wrap up Asian-inspired ingredients.

Soba noodles is an ingredient that it is worth adding to the store cupboard. They are lower in calories than wheat pasta and have a lovely nutty taste. They are also full of manganese, which helps to support the metabolism, vital for weight loss.

Ingredients (makes 3 wraps)

- 3 romaine lettuce leaves
- 3 x 1oz slice lean roast beef
- 1/4 cup sliced carrot
- 1/4 cup snow peas
- 1/4 cup broccoli florets

- 1/3 cup cooked soba noodles
- 1/4 cup chopped cilantro
- 1 tablespoon chopped peanuts
- 2 tablespoons rice wine vinegar
- 1/2 teaspoon chili paste
- 1 teaspoon sesame oil
- Juice from 1/2 lime
- PLUS 1 portion fruit

Method

1. Whisk together the rice wine vinegar, chili paste, 1 teaspoon sesame oil, lime juice and a dash of soy sauce.

2. Mix in the carrot, snow peas, chopped cilantro, and broccoli florets.

3. Add the cooked soba noodles and chopped peanuts, tossing all the ingredients to coat them all thoroughly.

4. Divide the mixture into three portions and place each on 1 romaine lettuce leaf topped with a 1-ounce slice of lean roast beef.

5. Roll the filled leaved into wraps and eat.

Chicken and Vegetable Soup

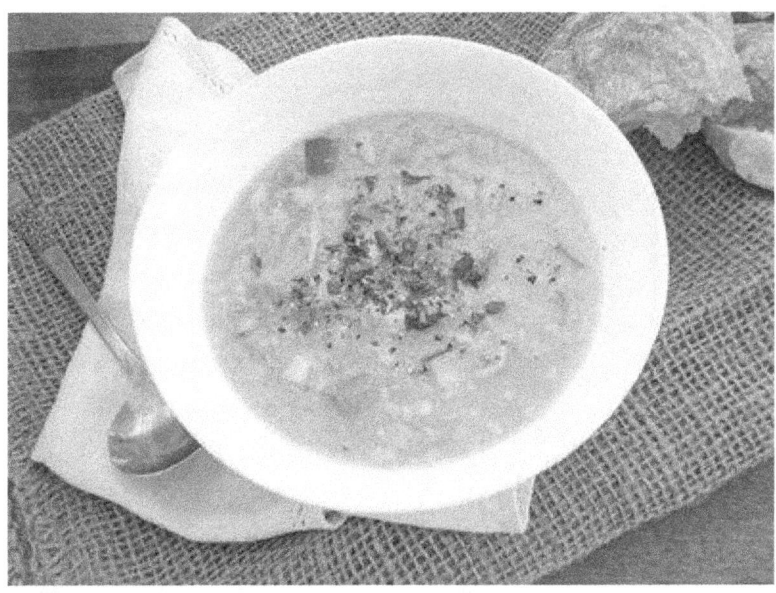

A wonderful, warming, hearty recipe for when you have time to cook something with love – it is a good recipe for a leisurely Saturday afternoon, for example. The lean chicken is very tasty and an excellent source of protein.

This makes several portions of soup, but soup always tastes better when made in large batches. You can share it with friends and family, but it also freezes well so you can make the soup and keep the rest for more deliciously healthy lunches or supper following the 17-Day Slim Down.

Ingredients

- 2 large carrots (chopped)
- 2 large leeks (trimmed and finely sliced)

- 2 corn on the cobs (corn kernels cut off)
- A small handful parsley (finely chopped)

For the stock

- 1 leek (cut into chunks)
- 2 carrots (thickly sliced)
- 2 bay leaves
- 6 black peppercorns
- A few parsley stalks
- 4 celery sticks (roughly chopped)
- 2 tbsp fat-free vegetable bouillon or 1 vegetable stock cube
- 1.3kg chicken (skinned)

Method

1. Put all the stock ingredients and the chicken in a very large saucepan, then cover everything with about 3 litres cold water.

2. Bring to the boil, then turn it down to a simmer and cook for 1 hr-1½ hrs, until the chicken is cooked through, being sure to skim off any froth or fat every 20 mins or so. Remove the chicken to a plate to cool.

3. Strain the stock through a sieve, skimming off as much fat as you can – there should not be too much as the chicken is skinless.

4. Put the stock back in, then simmer on a high heat until reduced down to about 2 litres in total. Add the carrots and leeks, then simmer for 10 mins.

5. While it is simmering, shred the meat from the chicken and discard the skin and bones. Add the chicken back to the pan, along with the sweetcorn.

6. After a few minutes when the corn is cooked through, ladle your soup into a large bowl and sprinkle it with the parsley. Leave the rest to cool so you can freeze it later.

Garden of Delight Salad

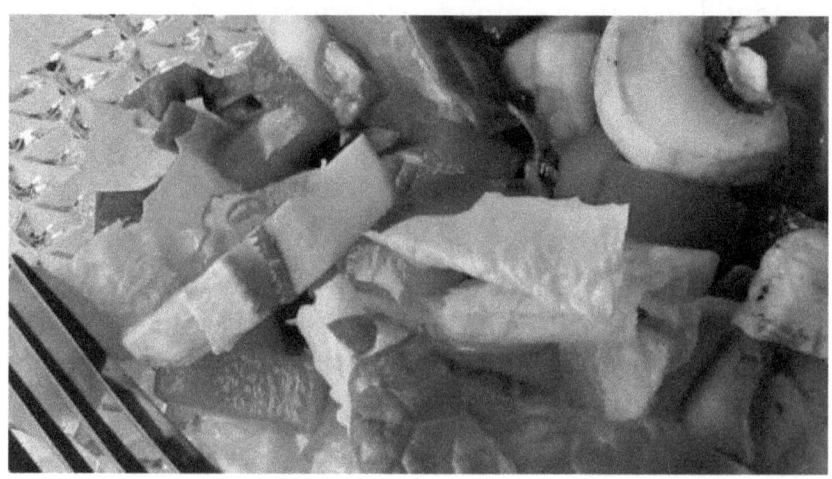

A super-simple, fresh and nutritious dish. The crisp iceberg lettuce makes the whole dish both filling and refreshing.

Use a really good quality thin ham, which will have had minimal additives or processing, just giving you some really tasty protein.

Also, don't be tempted to skimp on the beetroot – it really is a major superfood. Beetroot is packed with antioxidants, plus natural nitrates which permit more oxygen to flow in your blood and can improve performance in exercise.

Don't forget, since you are also doing your cardio and toning exercises as part of this diet plan, the foods we have selected are designed to be balanced and to ensure you have enough energy to work that body.

Ingredients

- 50g frozen peas
- 1 small beetroot (roughly diced)
- 1 tbsp fat-free Greek yogurt
- 1 tsp horseradish sauce
- ¼ iceberg lettuce (shredded)
- 50g thin sliced ham (cut into strips)

Method

1. Pour boiling water over the peas and leave for 2 mins, then drain well. Tip the peas and beetroot into a bowl and mix well.

2. Mix the yogurt with the horseradish, then add about 1 tbsp water to make a dressing.

3. Pile the lettuce into a bowl, then spoon over the beetroot mix. Thinly drizzle the dressing over the salad and top with ham. Welcome to the Garden of Delight!

Wheat Berry Salad

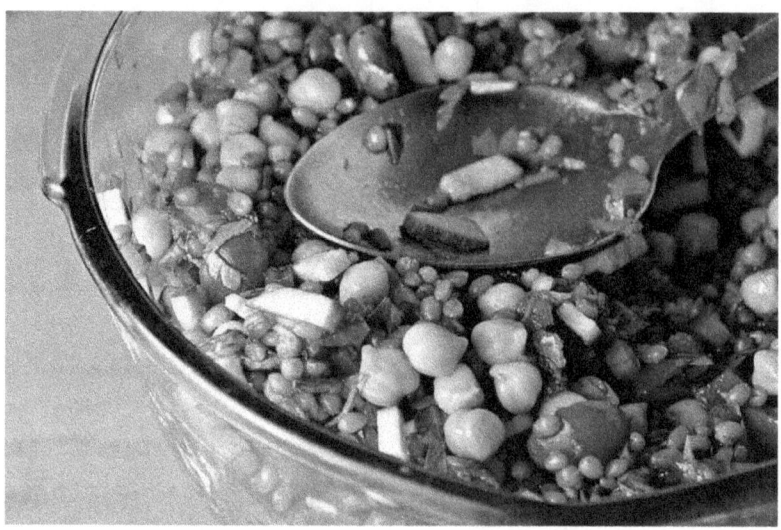

This is another good one for the weekend or for when you are feeling organized, as you need to let the wheat berries soak overnight.

Wheat berries, are essentially a whole kernel of wheat which includes the bran, wheat germ and endosperm. This is a superb whole food which provides exactly the kind of healthy fiber that will do your body go on the 17-Day Slim Down.

Plus, there is a lot of protein packed into your wheat berries, along with a bonanza of B vitamins. This makes each nutty little grain an amazing nutritional powerhouse – so stock up!

Ingredients

- ¾ cup wheat berries
- 1 cup chopped English cucumber

- ½ cup chopped arugula
- 1 tbsp fresh flat-leaf parsley (chopped)
- 1 cup cherry tomatoes (halved)
- 1 tsp grated lemon rind
- Juice of half a lemon
- Pinch of salt and freshly ground black pepper
- ½ tbsp extra-virgin olive oil
- 1oz reduced-fat goat's cheese

Method

1. The night before you want to make this dish, place the wheat berries in a medium bowl; cover with water to about 2 inches above the wheat berries. Cover and let stand for approximately 8 hours, draining the next morning.

2. Place the soaked wheat berries in a medium saucepan; cover with water to until it reaches 2 inches above the wheat berries. Bring to a boil, reduce heat, and cook for 1 hour or until tender.

3. Drain and rinse with cold water. Place the well-drained wheat berries into a bowl with the cucumber, tomatoes, arugula and parsley.

4. Combine the lemon rind, juice seasoning and oil in another small bowl and whisk into a dressing with a fork. Drizzle the dressing over the salad and toss well to coat all the ingredients.

5. Crumble in the reduced-fat goat's cheese and toss it again. Let the mixture stand for at least 30 minutes serve at room temperature.

Peachy Chicken Couscous

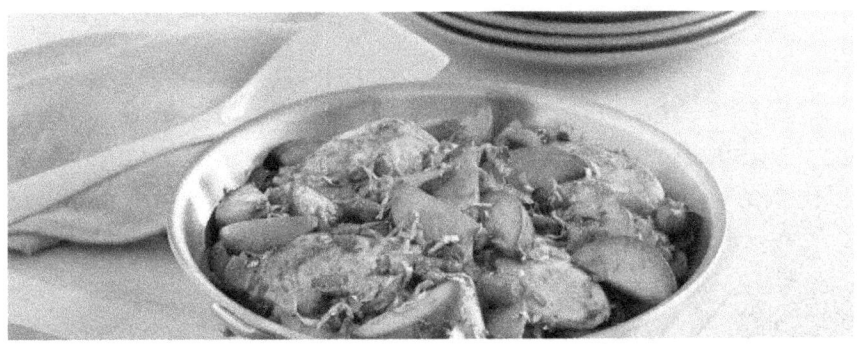

This is a super-tasty dish with the unusual addition of fresh peach to give you a great combination of flavors.

Whole-wheat couscous is a great grain for dieters when eaten in moderation. It is a relatively low-calorie carbohydrate and a little goes a long way, so you will feel well-fed and ready for an active afternoon.

Ingredients

- 90g cooked skinless boneless chicken breast (cut into bite size pieces)
- 75ml hot chicken stock
- 50g dried couscous
- Grated rind and juice of ¼ lemon
- 1 tbsp fresh cilantro (chopped)
- 1 peach (stoned and chopped)
- 4 cherry tomatoes (halved)
- 1 tbsp chives (chopped)
- A pinch of salt and freshly ground black pepper

Method

1. Heat the chicken stock in a pan.

2. In a large bowl, place the dry Couscous and pour the chicken stock over it. Add the lemon rind, juice and half the cilantro, then cover the bowl with cling film and leave it all to stand for 5 minutes.

3. When the time is up, fluff up the Couscous with a fork, put it into a serving dish and then leave it to cool completely.

4. When it is cool, stir in the chopped peach, tomatoes and chives. Season to taste.

5. Stir in the chicken and then scatter over the remaining cilantro. Ready to serve.

Chapter 11

Dinner Options

For many people, despite what nutritionists say about the importance of eating a good breakfast, dinner is the main meal of the day and the one they look forward to the most.

When we try to lose weight, we don't change overnight. It is therefore important to recognize the fact that we still love our food and don't want to feel deprived.

On the contrary, during the 17-Day Slim Down you have great meals to look forward to for 17 days in row!

The dinners in the following chapter are all well-balanced and interesting, with diverse flavors.

There are lots of vegetables and plenty of fiber added to sensible portions of meat and fish, with light helpings of wholegrain carbohydrates... all of which go to make a great healthy supper.

Nothing faddy, or over-the-top, just the best possible kinds of real food.

Remember, you don't strictly have to try all 17 dinner recipes during the Slim Down, you can simply repeat certain favorites if you prefer, but do try to keep a variety as that way you will enjoy a greater range of vital nutrients.

Also, we have taken a truly practical approach and given you recipes that serve at least 4 people and dinner is the meal when most people sit down together.

You can reduce the ingredients down for one, or simply enjoy trying out these recipes with family and friends – they are certainly good enough to share!

Charred Steak with Tomatillos

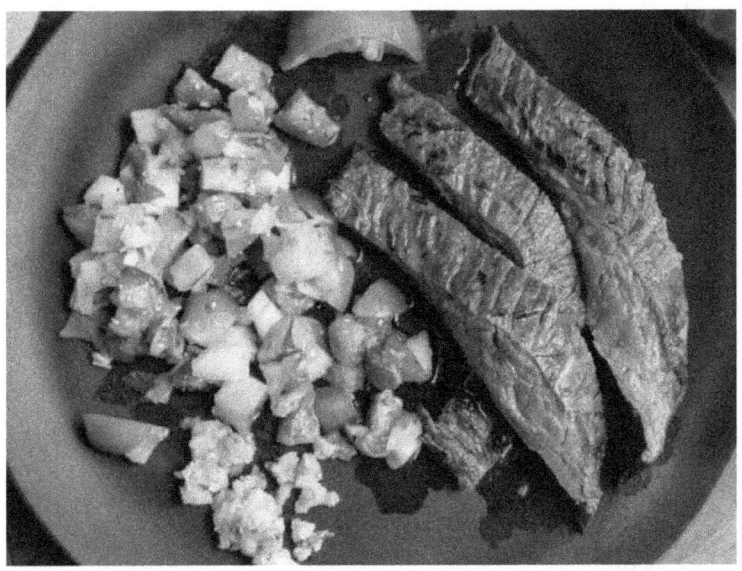

Many people worry that they will have to go without red meat when they are trying to lose weight. No such thing! The most important factors to consider if you are going to eat meat is the leanness of the cut and the amount of meat. Small amounts of meat with no excess fat will provide you with protein, iron, energy and possibly also a boost to your mood and morale.

The wonderful thing about this recipe is that it contrasts delicious strips of charred steak with fresh, fruity tomatillos. So good you can serve it up to dinner guests, at any time of year.

Ingredients (makes 4 portions)

- 1lb skirt steak (trimmed of all excess fat)
- 1 small chili

- 3 tbsp chopped fresh oregano (divided)
- 2 tbsp fresh lime juice (divided)
- 1 tbsp olive oil
- 1 1/2 tsp ground cumin (divided)
- 8 garlic cloves (divided)
- 8 ounces cherry tomatoes
- 1 tsp salt (divided)
- 3/4 tsp freshly ground black pepper (divided)
- 2 tbsp chopped fresh cilantro
- Low-calorie cooking spray

Method

1. Finely chop the chili and mince 4 garlic gloves. Combine the chili and minced garlic with 1 tablespoon oregano, 1 tablespoon lime juice, the oil and 1 teaspoon cumin in a zip-top plastic bag.

2. Add the steak to the bag, seal and then shake to coat. Refrigerate for 1 hour. Preheat oven to 450°.

3. Crush remaining 4 garlic cloves. Arrange crushed garlic over the tomatillos in a single layer on a baking sheet coated with cooking spray and lightly mist with some more cooking spray.

4. Bake at 450° for 20 minutes or until charred. Combine tomatillo mixture, remaining 2 tablespoons oregano, remaining 1 tablespoon juice, remaining 1/2 teaspoon cumin, 1/2 teaspoon salt and 1/4 teaspoon pepper in a blender and whizz up until it forms a smooth sauce.

5. Preheat the grill to high heat. Remove the steak from the bag; sprinkle both sides of steak evenly with remaining 1/2 teaspoon salt and remaining 1/2 teaspoon pepper.

6. Place steak on grill rack coated with cooking spray. Grill 2 minutes on each side or until the meat is done as you like it best. Let steak stand 10 minutes.

7. To serve, cut steak diagonally across grain into thin slices. Place 3 ounces steak on each of 4 plates. Top each serving with about 3 tablespoons sauce; sprinkle each serving with 1 ½ teaspoons cilantro.

Mediterranean Fish Hotpots

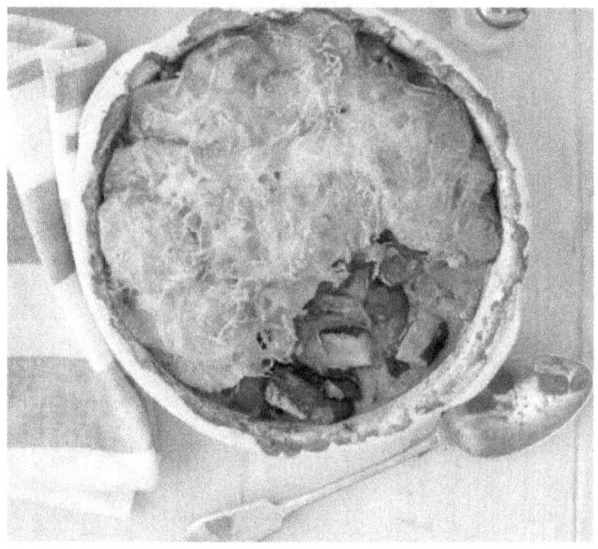

This has to be a number one dinner party dish for fish lovers everywhere! Hot and delicious pie dishes are filled with an unctuous fish and tomato sauce, for maximum flavor and low-calorie health benefits.

The white fish in this recipe is a primary source of super-lean protein, vitamin B12, iodine and selenium plus many more nutrients.

The tomato sauce is rich in lycopene, which can help prevent some cancers, diabetes and heart disease. It can also boost sperm production in men, prevent age-related deterioration of the skin, bones and eyes and limit sun damage. That's some sauce!

Specifically, in terms of weight loss, fish is a food that gives some of the best nutrient loads for relatively calories, so eat up without guilt and invite a few friends (or freeze the spares for another time)!

Ingredients (makes 6 hotpots)

- 3 tbsp olive oil
- 1 fennel bulb (trimmed and thinly sliced)
- 3 large garlic cloves (thinly sliced)
- 1 heaped tsp coriander seeds (lightly crushed)
- 2 x 400g cans chopped tomatoes with herbs
- 2 tbsp tomato purée
- A large pinch of saffron
- 1 bay leaf
- 1 tbsp fresh lemon juice
- 1 generous bunch of flat-leaf parsley (leaves roughly chopped)
- 900g mixed skinless white fish fillets, (cod, halibut etc) cut into large bite size chunks
- 350g raw peeled king prawns
- 75g finely grated parmesan
- 50g coarse dried whole-wheat breadcrumbs
- Green salad of lettuce leaves and cucumber (to serve)

Method

1. Heat the olive oil in a large nonstick pan and gently fry the fennel, garlic and coriander seeds for 15 mins, stirring regularly until the vegetables are softened and lightly colored.

2. Pour in the tomatoes and ass tomato purée, saffron and bay leaf. Season, stir and bring to a gentle simmer.

3. Cook the sauce for about 15 mins, stirring occasionally, until thick. Heat oven to 220C/200C fan/gas 7.

4. Stir the lemon juice and most of the parsley into the tomato sauce, place the raw fish pieces and prawns on top and stir well.

5. Cover tightly with a lid and simmer gently over a medium heat for 4-5 mins or until the fish is almost cooked. Stir a couple of times as the fish cooks, taking care not to let it break up.

6. Ladle the hot tomato and fish mixture into 6 individual pie dishes – they will each need to hold around 350ml.

7. Mix the cheese, Whole-wheat breadcrumbs, remaining parsley and a little ground black pepper together and sprinkle over the top.

8. Bake on a baking tray for 20 mins or until the pies are golden brown and bubbling. Serve with the fresh green salad on the side.

Fruity Wholegrain Chicken Salad

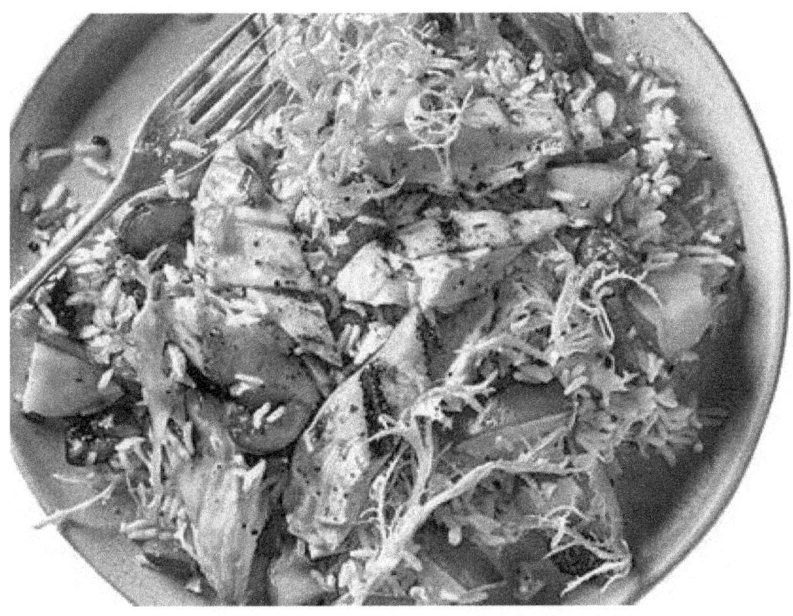

This wholesome dish is every bit as delicious as it sounds.

Chicken and brown rice is an outstanding combination, all lifted by the fruity and citrus accents and the refreshing torn mint. Brown rice is wonderful for your health.

It is a whole grain, which is very high in fiber and rich in selenium which reduces the risk for developing cancer, heart disease and arthritis. It is also rich in antioxidants, manganese and naturally occurring oils.

Plus, brown rice has been proven to promote weight loss as it supports the digestive system and helps it work at its peak.

Add to that all the vitamins and minerals with the fruit and nuts and a lot of lean protein and you have a really great, filling and nutritious dieting dish.

Ingredients (serves 4)

- 4 x 6oz. skinless, boneless chicken breast halves (trimmed)
- 2 cups cooked brown rice (cooled)
- 1 1/2 cups pitted (coarsely chopped nectarines)
- 1 cup coarsely chopped pitted fresh cherries
- 1/4 cup dry-roasted almonds (chopped)
- 3 tbsp torn mint
- 1 tsp grated lemon rind
- 2 tsp fresh lemon juice
- 2 tsp dijon mustard
- A large pinch of salt
- A pinch of black pepper
- 2 tbsp olive oil
- Low-calorie cooking spray

Method

1. Preheat the grill to medium-high heat.

2. Sprinkle both sides of chicken evenly with the salt and pepper. Place chicken on a grill rack coated with the low-calorie cooking spray; grill for 5 minutes on each side or until done.

3. Let the chicken stand for 5 minutes, then chop it into chunky bite size pieces.

4. Combine the oil, lemon rind and juice, and mustard in a large bowl, whipping it up well with a whisk.

5. Finally, add the chopped chicken, cooked brown rice, nectarines, cherries, almonds and torn fresh mint to the same bowl; toss well and serve.

Asian Salmon with Sugar Snap Salad

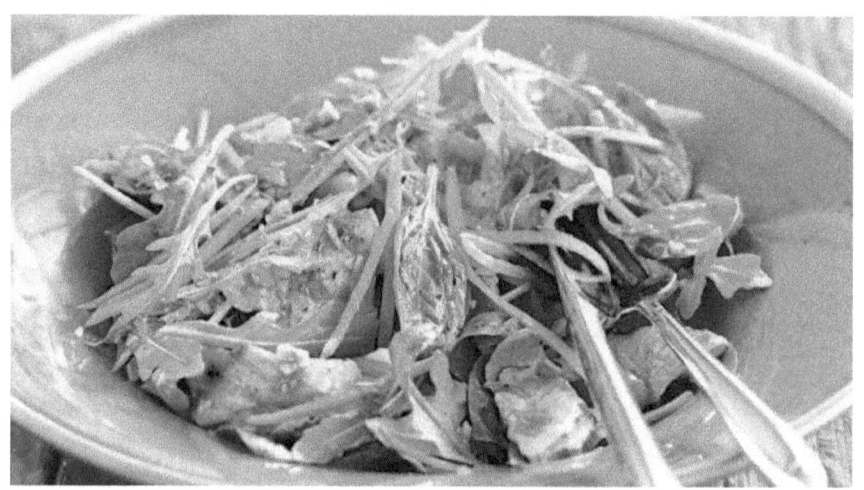

There are superfoods and then there are super-fish!

Salmon is an excellent oily fish and one that nutritionists recommend we should eat regularly.

It is brimming with omega-3 fatty acids, which is excellent for the brain, heart, joints and general health. It is also a fantastic source of high-quality protein, vitamins and minerals, including potassium, selenium and vitamin B12.

All this, for very few calories.

Ingredients (serves 4)

- 4 x 6oz fresh wild Alaskan salmon fillets
- 2 tbsp dark sesame oil (divided)

- 3 garlic cloves (crushed)
- A thumb-sized piece of fresh ginger (peeled)
- 2 tbsp fresh lime juice
- 2 tbsp lower-sodium soy sauce
- 1 tsp honey
- 1 small red chili (chopped)
- 2 cups sugar snap peas
- 1/2 cup grated radishes
- 2 teaspoons rice vinegar
- A good pinch of salt
- Low-calorie cooking spray

Method

1. Preheat the grill to high heat. Combine 1 tablespoon sesame oil, the garlic and the ginger in a mini food processor; pulse until finely chopped.

2. Add the lime juice, soy sauce, honey and chili then pulse to combine.

3. Place salmon fillets on a grill rack coated with the low-calorie cooking spray. Brush the surface of all the salmon with half of the sauce.

4. Grill salmon for 10 minutes then brush with remaining sauce. Grill an additional 10 minutes or until it is done to the degree that you like best.

5. Meanwhile, slice up the sugar peas and radishes.

6. Combine the vinegar and the remaining 1 tablespoon of oil, beating it with a fork so that it forms an emulsion.

7. Drizzle the dressing over the pea salad. Sprinkle with salt and lightly toss. Serve with the salmon.

Hoisin Pork Balls in Chinese Vegetable Broth

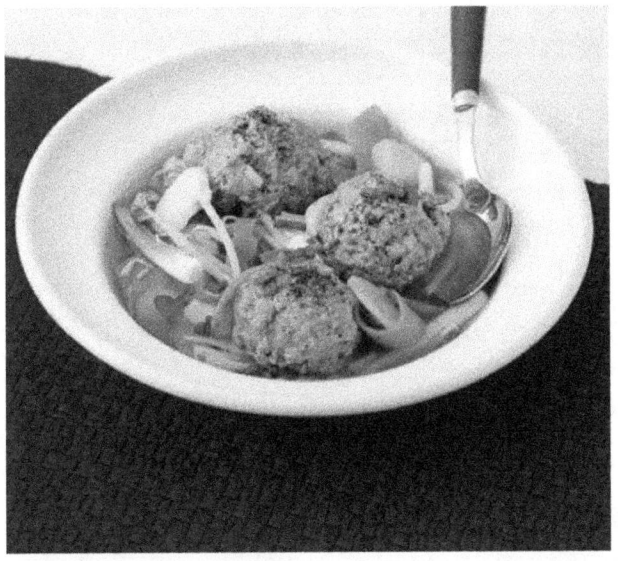

Pork can sometimes get a bad press among people who are trying to lose weight. After all, so many cuts of this popular red meat are too full of fat to enjoy during a weight loss regime – unsurprisingly this recipe does not feature belly pork.

However, you might be surprised at how easy it is to make the most of lean, low-fat pork. Either find your own top quality pork, which has been thoroughly trimmed and features no excess fat, or buy a ready-trimmed pack of lean pork mince.

It is worth the effort to find the leanest pork that mince you can, it can mean the difference of 100s of calories – 100g lean minced pork is just 164 calories – 100g pure pork fat is 900 calories... you do the math!

However, no fat NEVER has to mean no flavor. The pork balls make the most of this delicious meat by layering on the Asian flavors, all set off perfectly by the Chinese vegetables. Enjoy!

Ingredients (serves 4)

- 500g lean pork mince
- 2 tbsp soy sauce
- 2 tbsp cornflour
- 1 tsp Chinese five-spice powder
- 225g can water chestnuts, drained, half finely chopped, half sliced
- 500ml chicken stock
- 3 tbsp hoisin sauce
- thumb-sized piece ginger (shredded)
- 2 large carrots, shaved into strips with a potato peeler
- 8 Chinese leaves (thick part sliced, leaves shredded)
- 300g pack beansprouts
- A few very finely chopped chives to serve.

Method

1. Put the mince in a bowl with the soy sauce, corn flour, five-spice, chopped water chestnuts and some black pepper.

2. Work all these ingredients together in the bowl, then shape into 12 good-sized meatballs.

3. Pour the chicken stock into a wide, deep pan and stir in the hoisin and ginger. Add the meatballs, then cover and poach for 5 mins.

4. Drop in the carrots, Chinese leaves, beansprouts and the sliced water chestnuts, then put on the lid and simmer for 5 mins.

5. Ladle into bowls, then serve with a scattering of chopped chives.

Roast Snapper with Mediterranean Sauce

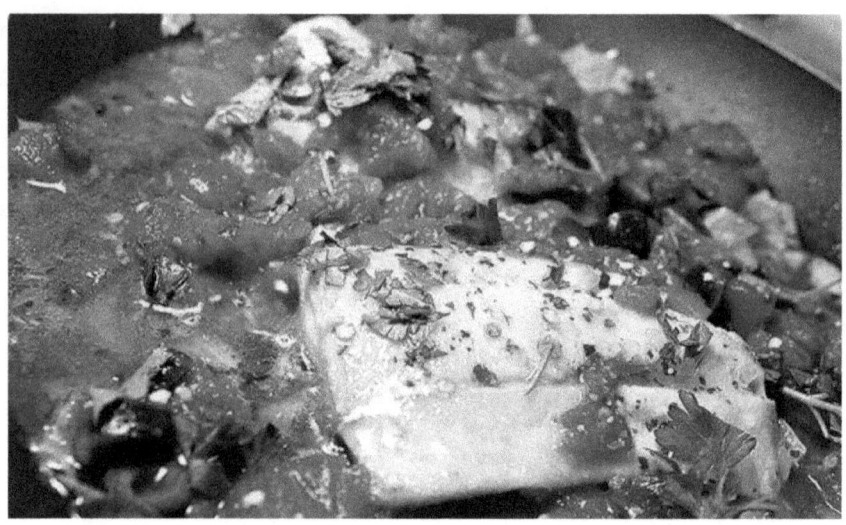

The wild-caught yellowtail snapper in this delicious dish is a real low-calorie treat. Yellowtail snapper makes a low-calorie, high protein, high-flavor star of the show.

It tastes especially good when cooked with a little canola oil, which has the lowest level of saturated fat of all cooking oils.

Ingredients (serves 4)

- 4 x 6oz yellowtail snapper fillets (skin on)
- 2 cups chopped seeded plum tomato
- 1 1/2 tbsp capers
- 1 tbsp dijon mustard
- 3 garlic cloves (minced)
- 1 1/2 tbsp chopped fresh flat-leaf parsley

- 1 1/2 tbsp minced fresh chives
- 1 tbsp minced fresh tarragon
- 1 1/2 tbsp olive oil
- 1 tbsp canola oil
- A large pinch of freshly ground black pepper (divided)
- A pinch of salt

Method

1. Heat the olive oil in a medium skillet over medium-high heat. Add the tomato to pan and cook for 5 minutes, stirring frequently.

2. Stir in the capers, Dijon mustard and minced garlic, allow to simmer for 3 minutes or until slightly thickened, stirring occasionally.

3. Remove from heat and stir in the parsley, chives, tarragon, salt and black pepper. Cover to keep warm.

4. Heat the canola oil in a large nonstick skillet over medium-high heat. Season the snapper lightly with salt and black pepper and add it to the pan, skin side down.

5. Cook for 3 minutes or until skin is browned, the turn the fish over; cook for a further 3 minutes or until it is as done as you like. Serve the fish with the sauce.

Turkey with Vegetable Soba Noodles

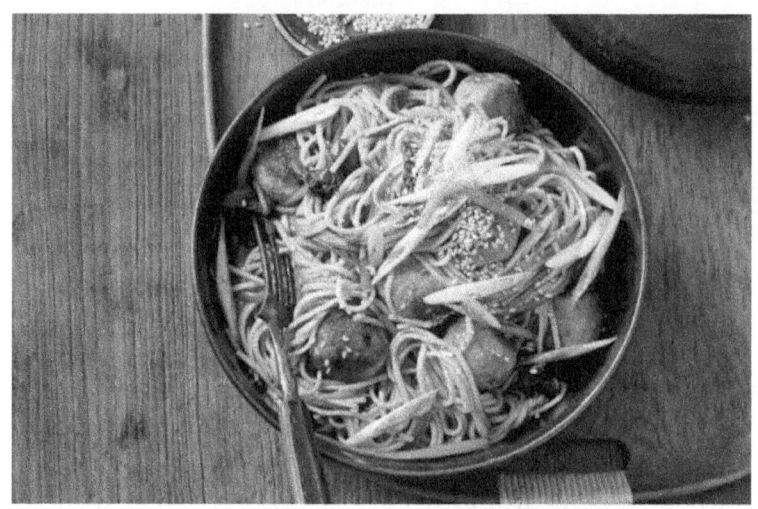

Turkey is not just for Christmas. This great white meat is actually even better for weight loss than chicken. A 3oz skinless turkey breast has only 90 calories and 1g fat, whereas a skinless chicken breast of the same size contains 165 calories and 5g fat.

So if you love the taste of turkey, don't hold back – make it your favorite meat. You can even use it to replace other meats in some of the other recipes in this book (just don't let this virtually fat-free protein dry out) and it you can enjoy it all year round.

Ingredients (serves 4)

- 3 x 4oz turkey (breast tenderloin steaks)
- 6 oz soba noodles (100% whole-grain, dried)

- 2 tsp light olive oil
- 2 cups sugar snap peas
- 1 cup carrots (julienned)
- 1 cup zucchini (julienned)
- 1 teaspoon sesame oil
- 1/2 cup plum sauce

Method

1. Cook soba noodles according to the directions on the packet and then drain. Return them to the saucepan, cover and keep warm.

2. Meanwhile, pour the olive oil into a wok or large skillet and heat it over a medium-high heat.

3. Stir-fry snap peas, carrots and zucchini in hot oil for 2 minutes or until vegetables are crisp-tender. Remove vegetables from wok.

4. Add turkey and sesame oil to the hot wok. Stir-fry for 3 to 4 minutes or until turkey is tender and no longer pink.

5. Add the plum sauce, stir and add the cooked vegetables back to the wok; stir to coat ingredients with sauce. Heat through. Serve immediately over the warm soba noodles.

Seared Scallops with Asian Citrus Salad

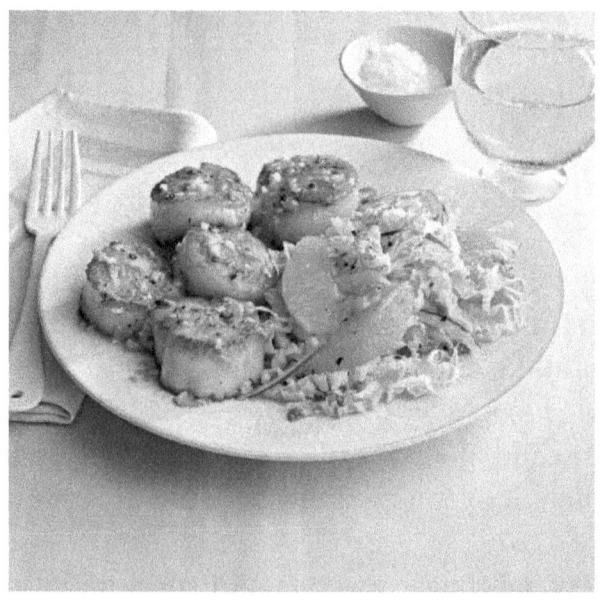

This wonderful recipe manages to be both sweet and savory, filling and light, exotic and good for every day, luxurious and yet great for weight loss. Scallop are a perennial seafood favorite and with good reason. They are full of vitamin B12, iodine, phosphorous and much more, yet low in calories and if you love food from the briny deep they taste absolutely fabulous.

Ingredients (serves 4)

- 16 sea scallops
- ¾ lb snow peas (halved lengthwise)
- 4 orange segments (peeled and broken into halves or thirds)

- 1 tbsp of very thinly sliced orange zest
- 1 cup couscous
- 1½ tbsp olive oil
- Salt and black pepper

Method

1. Cook the couscous according to the directions on the packet and cover it to keep it warm.

2. Meanwhile, heat about half of the oil in a large nonstick skillet over medium-high heat. Pat the scallops dry using paper towels and season with a pinched of salt and black pepper.

3. Cook the scallops until they are opaque throughout and light gold in color, just 2 to 3 minutes per side (any longer and they will become chewy). Transfer to a plate and cover.

4. Wipe out the skillet. Heat the remaining oil over a medium-high heat. Add the snow peas, orange zest, and another small pinch of salt and pepper.

5. Cook the pea and orange mixture, gently tossing the pan, until the snow peas are just tender, about 2 minutes. Remove the peas and zest from the heat, throw in the orange segments and stir.

6. Serve the citrus peas with the warm scallops and couscous.

Halibut with Lemon and Herbs

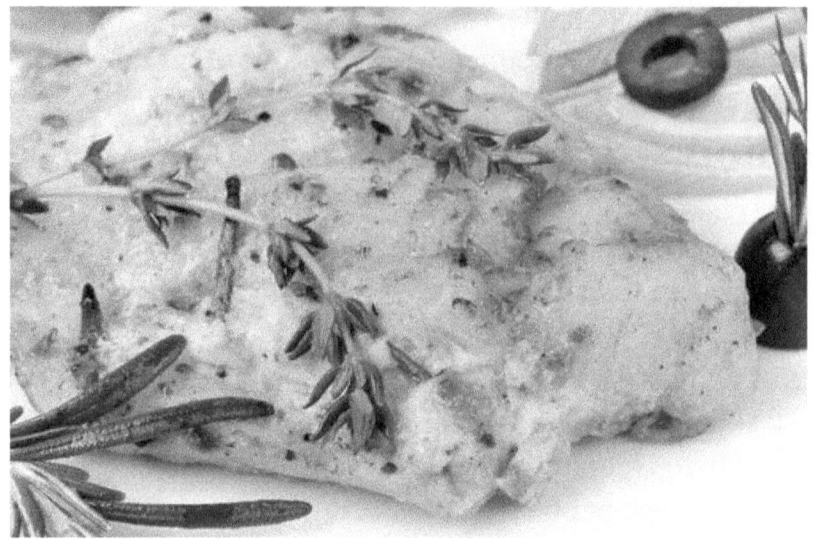

We have already explored the many benefits of eating freshly cooked white fish and halibut is another delicious example. This dish matches the fish with some fresh, zesty flavors in this nutrition-packed, vitamin C-rich herby sauce.

Ingredients

- 4 x 6oz halibut fillet
- 3 tbsp olive oil
- 1 1/2 tbsp chopped seeded jalapeno pepper
- 1 tbsp grated lemon rind
- 1 1/2 tbsp fresh lemon juice
- 4 tsp chopped fresh cilantro
- 4 tsp chopped fresh parsley
- 3 lemon sections (finely chopped)
- 6 cups water

- 1 parsley sprig
- 1 cilantro sprig
- A good pinch of pepper
- A good pinch of salt
- Salad leaves (to serve)

Method

1. First combine the chopped cilantro, chopped parsley, lemon juice, flesh and rind and the jalapeno and season lightly.

2. In a separate bowl, combine the water, parsley sprig, cilantro sprig remaining salt and pepper in a large skillet, then bring the poaching stock to a low simmer (180° to 190°).

3. Add the fish and cook it for 10 minutes or until it reaches the desired degree of doneness.

4. Remove fish from pan with a slotted spoon; drain on paper towels. Serve with the lemon and herb sauce and the salad leaves on the side.

Turkey Sausage and Kale Frittata Recipe

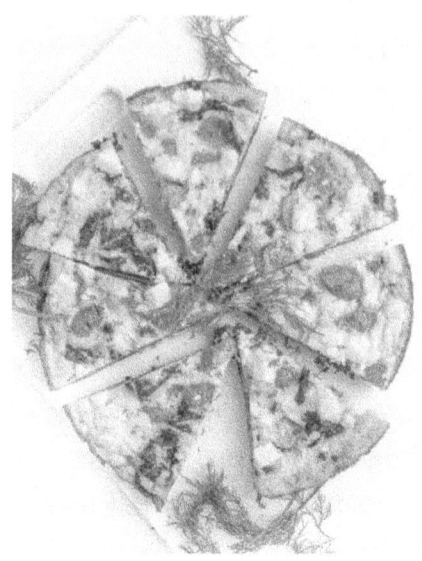

Sausage? On a 17-Day Slim Down? You bet! This is not just any sausage, this is super-lean turkey sausage, which has just a fraction of the fat but is just as tasty. It adds to the protein-power of this egg-laden suppertime treat.

Kale is an outstanding leafy green vegetable and a superfood in its own right. It is packed with fiber, calcium, and antioxidants, and it is super-healthy. Try not to overcook it to keep all those lovely nutrients in tip-top condition.

Ingredients

- 8 oz turkey sausage (removed from the casing and crumbled)
- 3 cups chopped kale

- 5 large eggs
- 1 cup egg whites
- 2 tablespoons chopped oregano
- 2 tablespoons olive oil (divided)
- 2 red potatoes (sliced thin)
- 3/4 cup cherry tomatoes (halved)
- 1 clove garlic (crushed)
- Salt and pepper to taste
- Salad leaves to serve

Method

1. Preheat the oven to 375° F.

2. In a large bowl, whisk together the first eggs, egg whites and oregano, lightly season with salt and pepper. Heat 1 tablespoon of olive oil in a 10-inch cast-iron skillet over medium-high heat.

3. Add the sausage and cook it until browned. Transfer it to a plate and set aside. Heat the remaining 1 tablespoon oil in the skillet over medium heat.

4. Place the potatoes in the skillet, cover, and cook, stirring occasionally, until tender but firm, for about 10 minutes.

5. Add the kale, tomatoes and garlic. Continue cooking for 3 minutes, until kale is wilted. Season with salt and pepper to taste.

6. Stir in the reserved sausage and pour in the egg mixture. Swirl the egg around gently to spread it over the ingredients, but do not stir.

7. Transfer the skillet to the oven and bake until set, about 15 minutes. Cut into 4 wedges and serve with green salad leaves on the side.

Chicken Kebabs with Mixed Med Veg

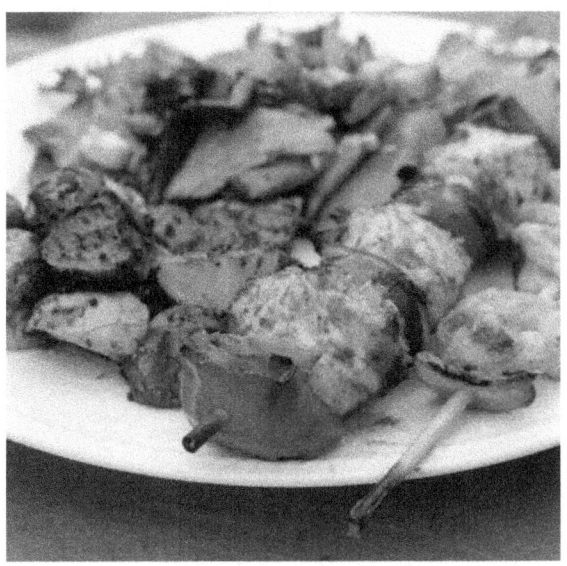

Ingredients

For the kebabs

- 4 chicken breasts (chopped into large bite-sized pieces)
- 2 cups medium mushrooms

For the sauce

- 2 cups cherry tomatoes
- 2 cloves garlic
- A few leaves of torn basil
- Salt and pepper

Plus

- 2 cups cooked pearl barley (kept warm)
- 3 cups chunky-cut vegetables (zucchini, carrots, beets)
- Low-calorie cooking spray

Method

1. Pre-heat the oven to 350°F. Roast the chunky cubes of vegetables in an oven tray, spraying them with a spritz of the low-calorie cooking spray. Let them start to caramelize nicely, which should take around 20-30 minutes.

2. At the same time, cook the 4 chicken kebabs. Feed the large cubes of chicken and the mushroom onto skewers and then spray them with low-calorie cooking spray. Place the kebabs on a grill pan which has also been misted with the low-calorie cooking spray.

3. While the kebabs and vegetables are cooking, make the sauce. Cut the cherry tomatoes in half and put in a warm skillet spritzed with low-calorie cooking spray. After 3 minutes crush in the garlic and stir.

4. When the tomatoes have fully softened, finish the sauce turning off the heat and adding in the torn basil.

5. When the chicken kebabs and vegetables are tender and cooked through, serve them with the warm pearl barley and a generous pouring of the tomato sauce.

Turkey Bolognaise

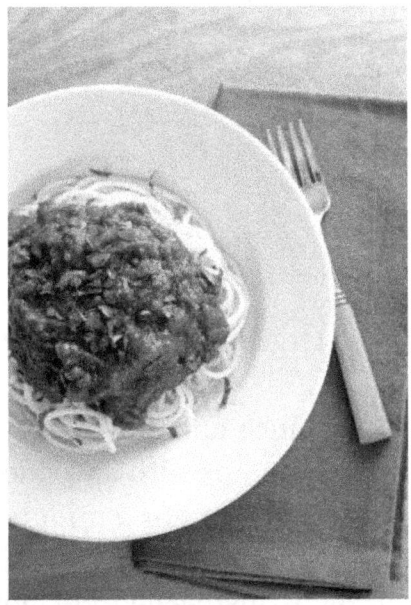

One of the great pleasures of going on the 17-Day Slim Down – besides watching all those unwanted pounds slip away – is discovering great new lighter alternatives to some favorite family recipes.

Bolognaise is the Italian sauce that everybody loves and this superb turkey version has just a fraction of the calories compared to the standard beef variety. Add to that the fact that is it is served with warm quinoa and not regular pasta and you can see why this is a fantastic, tasty option for slimmers!

Ingredients (serves 4)

- 2 cups lean turkey mince
- 2 cups cooked quinoa (kept warm)

- 2 x 400g cans chopped tomatoes
- 2 large carrots (diced)
- 1 clove of garlic
- A pinch of dried mixed herbs
- 2 tsp olive oil for preparation
- Green salad leaves

Method

1. Heat the oil in a large skillet, on a medium-high heat.

2. Add the turkey mince and slowly fry it, taking care to break up any large lumps with a wooden spoon. Add the dried carrot and stir for a 1 or 2 minutes.

3. When the turkey is just sealed but not turning brown, add the chopped tomatoes to the pan.

4. Crush the garlic and add it to the turkey sauce, along with the herbs. Leave to simmer gently for 5 minutes or until the sauce begins to thicken.

5. Serve the sauce on a small bed of warm quinoa, with some green salad leaves on the side.

Rainbow Supper

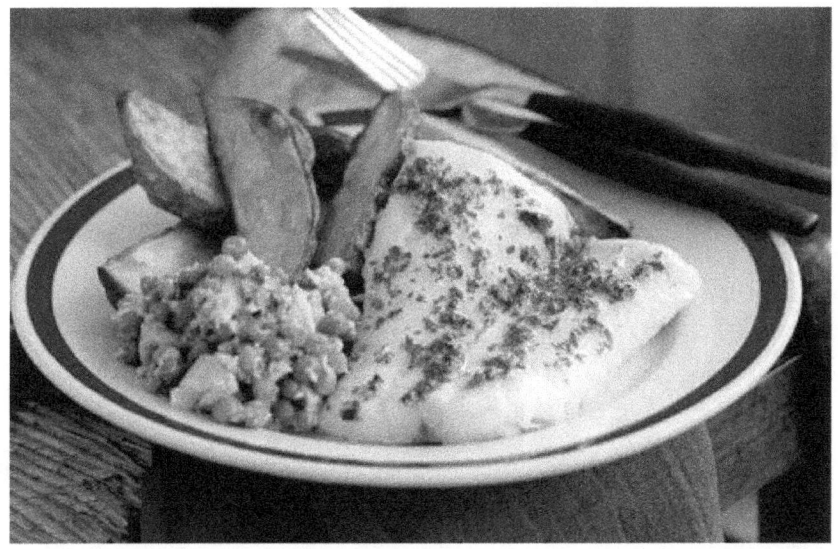

This highly nutritious supper has everything you need for a 17-Day Slim Down meal. The rainbow trout provides lean protein, vitamins and minerals, the sweet potato give some good carbs with plenty of fiber, as do the green beans and spinach.

Your rainbow supper makes a relaxing weekday meal that is so easy to make. Ideal for when you do want anything complicated and fancy kicking back with some

Ingredients (serves 4)

- 4 fillets of rainbow trout
- 4 medium sweet potatoes
- 4 tsp olive oil
- 4 tsp pesto
- 4 cups green beans

- 6 cups spinach
- A squeeze of lemon juice
- A pinch of black pepper
- A pinch of salt

Method

1. Pre-heat the oven to 350°F. Cover each of the sweet potatoes in oil, rubbing it into the skin. Sprinkle each potato with the salt and put in the oven for around 40 minutes or until sharp knife goes softly through them.

2. When it is 10 minutes until the potatoes are ready, put the rainbow trout fillets on the grill. Leave to cook for a few minutes until just done.

3. Drop the green beans and the spinach into separate pans of boiling water for 3 minutes.

4. When all the elements are ready, put the trout on plates and squeeze over a little fresh lemon juice. Drain the green vegetables and add to the plates.

5. Serve up a potato each, by splitting the top and topping each one with a little pesto sauce. It's all ready!

Squashed Chicken

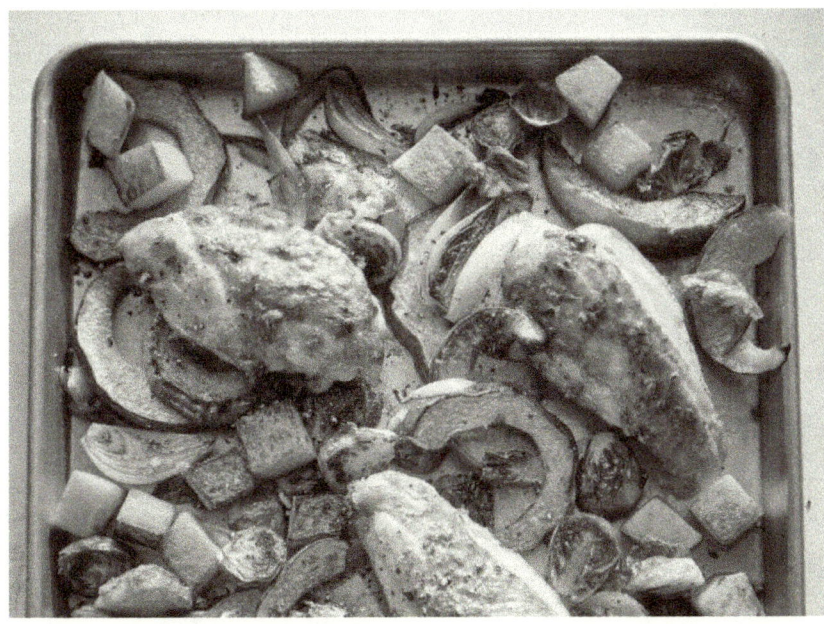

This recipe is not named after flattened poultry, but because it contains both butternut squash and gem squash. Both vegetables are a friend to anyone who is trying to lose weight.

Butternut squash boasts a lot of antioxidants and vitamins for very few calories. Gem squash is also low in calories and has a high water content so is great for when you are slimming down. It is also packed with carotene, ideal for warding off a wide range of diseases including heart disease.

Ingredients

- 4 skinless chicken breasts
- 2 butternut squashes (halved and de-seeded)
- 2 gem squashes halved and de-seeded

- 4 medium tomatoes (halved)
- 2 tbsp olive oil
- A pinch of cinnamon
- A large handful of torn fresh cilantro

Method

1. Preheat the oven to 350°F. Sprinkle the butternut squash with a little cinnamon. Place them, along with the gem squashes, on baking trays and drizzle all with half the oil. Leave them in the oven to roast.

2. After 20 minutes drizzle the chicken breasts with the remaining oil and place on another baking tray, along with the tomatoes, for at least 25 minutes.

3. When the chicken is done, remove everything from the oven. Take chunky scoops of butternut and gem squash with a spoon, pile them on each plate with the tomatoes and chicken and scatter plenty of fresh coriander over the dishes, then serve.

Whole-Wheat Crab Cakes

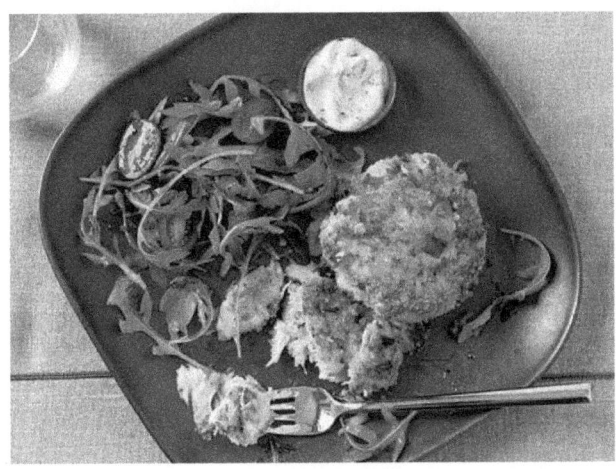

This is as healthy a version of crab cakes as you will ever find. Crab is a delicious seafood which is bursting with protein and full of omega-3 fatty acids. Better still, it is only 82 calories per 3 ounces and it tastes absolutely wonderful! This recipe ups the fiber content by using whole-wheat breadcrumbs and serving a fresh salad on the side. Don't skip the squeeze of lime as it brings out the crab flavor beautifully and adds a welcome dash of vitamin C.

Ingredients

To make 6 crab cakes

- 1lb crabmeat
- 1 egg (lightly beaten)
- ½ cup whole-wheat panko-style breadcrumbs
- ½ cup extra-light mayo
- 2 tbsp chives (finely chopped)

- 1 tbsp Dijon mustard
- 1 tbsp lemon juice
- 1 tsp celery seed
- ¼ tsp freshly ground pepper
- 4 dashes hot sauce
- 2 tablespoon canola olive oil

To serve

- 1 cucumber
- 2 handfuls of lettuce leaves
- 4 medium tomatoes
- 2 limes

Method

1. Mix the crab, egg, breadcrumbs, mayonnaise, chives, mustard, lemon juice, celery seed, pepper and hot sauce in a large bowl. Form the mixture into 6 patties.

2. Heat the canola oil in a large nonstick skillet over medium heat and cook the patties until golden brown, about 4 minutes per side.

3. While they are cooking, take a vegetable peeler and peel down the whole length of the cucumber to make thin ribbons. Pile onto the plate with torn lettuce leaves and wedges of the tomato.

4. Serve the crab cakes as soon as they are ready, with the side salad and ½ a lime to squeeze over your food.

Japanese Steak Stir Fry

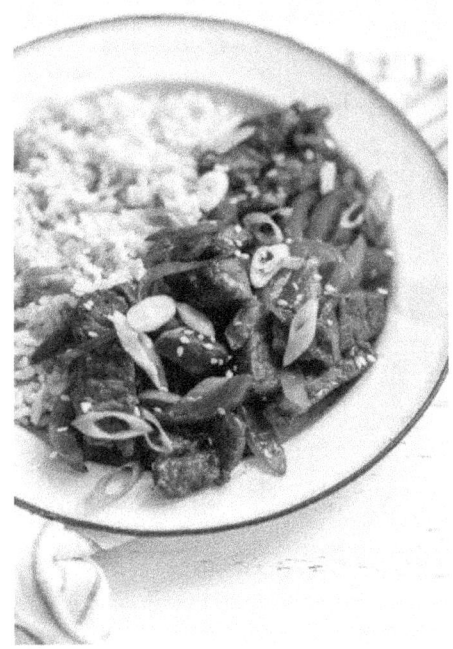

Choose the leanest cut of skirt steak that you can find for this enticing oriental recipe, which will fill you up with fresh flavors. Don't forget to add the cashews at the end – they are high in anti-oxidants and far lower in fat than many other types of nut.

Ingredients

- ½ lb skirt steak
- 2 garlic cloves (finely chopped)
- 2 tbsp lime juice
- 1 tsp olive oil
- 2 ½ cups diagonally cut asparagus
- 1 tbsp fresh ginger peeled and grated

- 1 tbsp low-sodium soy sauce
- 2 tsp sesame oil
- 1 tbsp lime juice
- 2 cups cooked brown rice
- ½ cup chopped fresh cilantro
- tbsp chopped cashews

Method

1. Cut steak crosswise into 1/4-inch-thick strips. Toss together with garlic, and 2 tablespoons lime juice; marinate the steak for 15 minutes.

2. Heat 1/2 teaspoon olive oil in a wok or nonstick skillet over medium-high heat.

3. Cook the steak with the marinade, stirring constantly, for 2-3 minutes or until medium-rare; transfer with slotted spoon to a large bowl, and set aside.

4. Add 1/2 teaspoon olive oil and asparagus to wok; cook, stirring, for about 4 minutes or until tender.

5. Put steak back into the wok. Add the ginger, soy sauce, sesame oil, and 1 tablespoon lime juice to wok and cook, stirring, for about 2 minutes or until heated through.

6. Add cooked brown rice to the wok and heat for 2 minutes. Divide the stir-fry among 4 plates, and scatter chopped cilantro and chopped cashews on top then serve.

Seasoned Pork with Kale

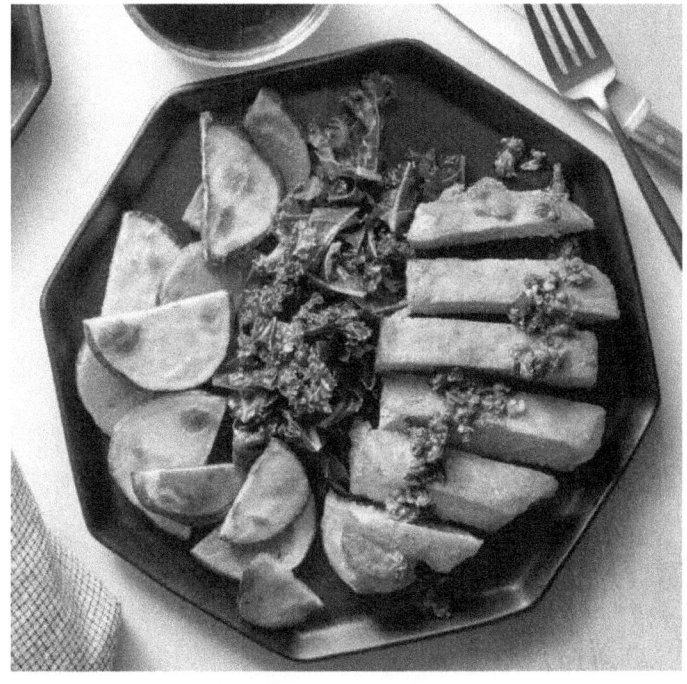

Pork tenderloin is typically wonderful in flavor and very lean. These seasonings blend together to make a terrific rub, which delivers a whole heap of vibrant added taste without piling on lots of unwanted calories. The meat goes perfectly with some freshly steamed kale and wholegrain rice.

Ingredients (serves 4)

- 1 1/4 pounds pork tenderloin
- 1 tsp garlic powder
- 1 tsp dried oregano
- 1 tsp ground cumin
- 1 tsp ground coriander

- 1 tsp dried thyme
- 1 tbsp olive oil
- 1 tsp minced garlic
- A large pinch of salt

To serve

- 12 large kale leaves (chopped)
- 2 cups wholegrain rice

Method

1. Preheat the oven to 450 degrees F. In separate bowl mix dry ingredients such as garlic powder, oregano, cumin, coriander, thyme and salt. Stir the mixture with a fork until all the ingredients are well combined and they form a seasoning.

2. Put a pan of water on another ring and bring it to the boil. Sprinkle the seasoning rub over the tenderloin with a dry hand, then rub the pork with the seasoning over both sides of the meat, pressing gently so the seasoning sticks well to the surface of the tenderloin.

3. In a large skillet over medium-high heat, add the olive oil and heat. Add the minced garlic and sauté, stirring, for 1 minute.

4. Add the tenderloin in the pan and brown it to seal in the juices for about 10 minutes, searing each side and carefully using tongs to turn the meat.

5. When the water is boiling, put in the cups of wholegrain rice and leave to cook for 25 minutes.

6. Meanwhile, transfer the meat to a roasting pan and bake for 20 minutes. While the pork is cooking, steam the kale for 4 minutes.

7. When the tenderloin is ready, slice it into thick medallions and serve with the kale and rice.

Chapter 12

Snacking Options

Your main meals will feel you up and give you the perfect balance of nutrition. However, you still need to enjoy a daily snack to keep your metabolism running at its best.

Another reason why this weight loss plan is so great – the delicious, nutritious daily snacks!

Pick one of these 17 snacks each day and ideally enjoy it between lunch and dinner:

- 3 wholegrain crackers, lightly spread with a mixture of smoked mackerel, mashed with fat-free plain yoghurt and seasoned with pepper.

- Half a small whole-meal roll, toasted and topped with low-fat cottage cheese.

- 1 piece of fruit from the Fruit Portions list.

- 150ml fat-free plain yoghurt.

- Crudités – raw cucumber, carrot, celery and radish, as much as you like – with a tablespoon of reduced fat hummus as a dip.

- A nice hot bowl of organic miso soup – the packets are available from good health stores and supermarkets.

- A rye crispbread topped with a sliced tomato and a tablespoonful of low-fat cottage cheese.

- 5 spears of asparagus, drizzled with a very little olive oil, then roasted in a 350°F oven for a few minutes until just tender. Sprinkle with a little salt and eat as a great hot snack.

- Enjoy a bowl of quick vegetable broth. Boil a two bowlfuls of water. Toss in an organic chicken stock cube.

   Chop 1 large carrot, some broccoli florets, a few mushrooms and two celery stalks and them to the stock and simmer until tender and the stock has reduced a little. Season with pepper and any fresh herbs you have to hand, then serve.

- Have a roast cauliflower treat. Take 5-7 florets of cauliflower and drizzle them with light olive oil and sprinkle with a pinch of salt and pepper.

   Place in a roasting dish in an oven pre-heated to 350°F for 15-20 minutes or until they are lightly golden brown and tender. Eat immediately (mind your tongue)!

- Enjoy a super-healthy green smoothie. Blend a handful of kale, a few leaves of baby spinach, a cup of unsweetened coconut water, 1 green apple and a few cubes of ice. When it is blitzed and smooth, drink cold.

- Eat a large handful of super-antioxidant blueberries, topped with a tablespoon of thick, fat-free Greek yoghurt.

- Baked mushrooms – Take 2 large mushrooms, stuff them with cherry tomatoes, drizzle with oil and sprinkle with salt and pepper. Cook in a hot oven for 15-20 minutes until tender and the tomatoes are oozing juice, then eat.

- Try 2/3 of a tablespoon of mixed seeds that includes pumpkin, sesame, sunflower seeds and more for some delicious healthy fats.

- If you fancy a delicious sweet treat, try a vanilla and banana smoothie. Blend half a banana with ¼ cup on fat-free vanilla yogurt and a few cubes of ice for a gorgeous drink.

- Stuffed figs: take two small dried figs and stuff them with 1 tablespoon reduced-fat ricotta. Sprinkle with a little cinnamon and eat.

- Make some apple chips, with no added sugar. Preheat the oven to 200 F. Thinly slice two apples crosswise about 1/8-inch (2 mm) thick with a mandolin or sharp knife.

  Arrange apple slices in a single layer on baking sheets. Sprinkle 1 teaspoon of cinnamon evenly over apple slices. Bake for 2 hours or until apples are dry and crisp, then eat. They can also be made in larger batched and stored in an airtight container for up to 3 days.

Others who are considering purchasing this book would love to know what you think. If you could spare a few seconds, they would greatly appreciate reading an honest review from you. Simply visit the book page on Amazon.com.

Chapter 13

Accelerate the Weight Loss

So, you have everything you need to lose weight over the next 17 days… but maybe you still want more? As with any weight loss program, you can take the 17-Day Weight Loss plan to the max by taking note of a few little tips that will help to accelerate the weight loss:

Keep the carbs to a minimum

This is by no means a carb-free diet as we believe in the proven power of high-fiber wholegrains. However, you do not need to have too much of these filling starches.

If you would like to lose weight more quickly, then cut the portion size of the starchy carbs like wholegrain rice etc in half. You won't go hungry – just top up your plate with the lower-calorie green carbs like kale and spinach.

Keep your metabolism running well

Certain small daily changes to your routine can add up to a far more active metabolism. Do try to stay on the move, don't sit all day – get up stretch and walk around.

Check that you are taking 10,000 steps

This is the recommended number of steps that any person is supposed to take per day to remain fit and active. It is a great way of measuring whether you are moving around enough generally, in addition to your 17-minute exercises. If you fit in 10,000 steps as well, the weight will just drop off! To see whether you are on track you can...

Use an activity tracker

You must have seen these – at first glance they look like a watch but they are in fact a great bit of wearable tech. Activity trackers, like Garmin Vivofit, Microsoft Band or the FitBit can monitor all kinds of areas directly related to your health including the amount of exercise you take, the calories you burn, the speed you walk, the quality of your sleep... and yes, the amount of steps that you take every day.

Use this kind of gadget when you find it hard to keep tabs on just how much you are moving around. Also, think of the extra motivation that you will gain from learning how many calories you are burning.

You can sync these devices with apps like My Fitness Pal or similar, so that you can input what you eat – but that is not required for this 17-Day Slim Down. Simply use it to check you have hit the golden 10,000 steps and make it a healthy no-brainer.

Swap your Fruit Portions for Veg

Fruit is a natural miracle and we love it. Eaten as part of a healthy diet, it will fill you with vitamins and fiber, refresh you and help you lose weight.

However, there is no denying that fruit does contain natural sugars, in the form of fructose. This is a sugar that the body copes with well, but it means that gram for gram, a fruit is likely to be higher in calories than a green vegetable.

You will lose weight on the 17-Day Slim Down just as it is, and you will also enjoy the range of flavors. But if you want to take a slightly stricter approach which may help you shed a few more pounds, then try replacing some of the fruit portions with salad vegetables – celery sticks, for example, or an undressed watercress and cucumber salad, or a few radishes.

These have a high-water content, lots of fiber and a very low-calorie count. So, tuck in!

Chapter 14

After the 17 Days...

So, you have successfully completed the 17-Day Slim Down.

Congratulations!

You will be looking and feeling much fitter, slimmer and healthier all round.

Don't believe us? Well not only can you hop on the scales to check how many pounds you have lost, but we advise that you also take a celebratory 'After' selfie.

Remember the photo that you took at the start of the 17 days. Take one right now and compare and contrast.

Do you look different, perhaps a little less blurry around the edges? Leaner, meaner and more prepared for an active demanding life? Great!

But one still question remains... what happens now that the 17 days are up? The answer is, that's up to you!

You can stop the plan, although ideally you will carry on enjoying all the great benefits of this program by maintaining the key elements of the diet and exercise. As long as you continue to keep the calories low and the fiber and exercise levels high, you will not regain weight.

Better still, why not continue with the principles of the 17-Day Slim Down and, if you need to, continue to lose weight?

This is a diet that really does delivery the double-whammy – you can use it as a quick-fix to drop some unwanted pounds in the healthiest way possible, or you can adapt it into a longer-term plan.

To make sure that the weight stay off, remember the keep principles of the plan and stick with them – high fiber, high water, low calorie, low fat. Eat minimal processed food and get moving too. Stick with these key ideas and your body will keep on thanking you in return.

As your body continues to slim down after the 17 days, you may find you need even fewer carbs and can reduce the wholegrain rice, noodles or other carbohydrates by a third or even by half.

You may also wish to gradually reintroduce some of the eliminated foodstuffs, like onions, beans or cabbage, if you like them and they do not give you an adverse reaction.

You may want to change up the cardio exercises so that you get maximum variety – keep on burning more calories than you eat and you will continue to be in even more fabulous shape.

No need to stop doing the body transformation exercises either. If you want to stay in shape, keep on toning your abs, legs and butt with the suggested workouts, or add in new ones. Even if you need to slash the 17 minutes to 10, just do it!

Apart from that, just keep going! When you reach your ideal weight, don't go back to your 'old' ways, just slightly increase portion sizes and allow yourself a bit more flexibility and the occasional 'off-menu' treat – but do keep up the exercise.

You may be amazed at the amount of weight that you lose and keep off by continuing to enjoy this totally healthy, totally sustainable diet.

Chapter 15

Shopping List

Shopping List

Here is a shopping list that includes absolutely everything that crops up in the recipes and meal ideas that have been presented in the diet plan.

But first, when it comes to buying the food for your 17-Day Slim Down, a few quick tips:

Do take your time to read through all the recipes first and select the ones that you would like to try first. Then you can mark off the ingredients which go into your recipes of choice.

Depending on whether the food is fresh or not, e.g. whether it is a carrot or a packet of oats, you may not want to buy it all in advance to eat on Day 17, for example.

We would recommend selecting menus for up to 5 days and shopping accordingly every 5 days or so, just to make the shopping more manageable.

- alfalfa sprouts
- almonds dry-roasted
- apples (red and green)
- apple sauce (unsweetened)
- apricots
- arugula

- asparagus
- avocado
- banana
- basil (fresh)
- beansprouts
- beef (lean & sliced thinly)
- beetroot
- berries (mixed)
- blueberries
- bran flakes
- broccoli
- bulgur wheat
- butternut squash
- capers
- carrots (large)
- cashew nuts
- cauliflower
- celery
- cheddar cheese (reduced fat)
- Cherries
- cherry tomatoes
- chicken (skinless & fresh)
- chicken stock (organic)
- Chili (red)
- Chinese leaves
- chives (fresh)
- cilantro (fresh)
- coconut water
- corn on the cob
- cottage cheese (low-fat)
- couscous

- crabmeat (white and brown mixed)
- cranberries (dried)
- cranberry juice (no added sugar)
- cream cheese (reduced fat)
- eggs (large & organic)
- fennel
- feta cheese (low fat)
- figs (dried)
- garlic
- gem squash
- ginger (fresh)
- goat's cheese (reduced fat)
- grapefruit (pink)
- grapes
- green beans
- guava (large)
- halibut fillets
- ham (top quality & thinly sliced)
- honey (natural blossom variety)
- horseradish sauce (fresh)
- hummus (reduced fat)
- jalapeno
- kale
- king prawns (raw)
- kiwi fruit
- leeks
- lemons
- lettuce (iceberg)
- lettuce leaves (baby variety & mixed)
- lettuce (romaine)
- limes

- low-calorie cooking spray
- mackerel (smoked)
- mango
- mayo (extra-light)
- melon
- milk (fat-free)
- milk powder (nonfat)
- mint leaves (fresh)
- miso soup paste
- mozzarella (part-skim)
- muesli (low-fat)
- mushrooms (chestnut or button variety)
- oats
- olives (black)
- oranges
- orange juice
- oregano (fresh)
- parmesan
- parsley (flat-leaf & fresh)
- passion fruit
- pawpaw
- peach
- peanuts
- pear
- peas (frozen)
- pesto
- pineapple
- plums
- plum sauce
- pork mince
- pork tenderloin

- potatoes (red)
- prunes
- pumpkin seeds
- quinoa
- quinoa flakes
- radishes
- rainbow trout fillets
- raspberries
- rice, brown
- ricotta (low fat)
- rye bread
- rye crispbread
- salmon (fresh 5 oz. fillet)
- salmon (5 oz. can)
- salmon (smoked and thinly sliced)
- satsumas
- scallops
- seed bread
- seeds (mixed)
- shrimp (large & fresh)
- snow peas
- soba noodles
- spinach (baby leaves)
- squash (yellow)
- steak (skirt)
- strawberries
- sugar snap peas
- sunflower seeds
- sweet potatoes
- tarragon (fresh)
- tomatoes (chopped and canned)

- tomatoes (fresh)
- tomatoes (plum)
- tuna (canned in spring water)
- turkey breast tenderloin steaks
- turkey mince (fresh, or an organic turkey patty)
- turkey sausage
- vanilla extract
- walnuts
- water chestnuts
- watercress
- watermelon
- wheat berries
- wheat germ
- whole-wheat bread
- whole-wheat breadcrumbs
- whole-wheat burger bun
- whole-wheat crackers
- whole-wheat English muffins
- whole-wheat pita bread
- whole-wheat roll (small)
- whole-wheat sub roll
- whole-wheat tortillas (fat-free)
- whole-wheat wrap
- yellow squash
- yellowtail snapper fillets
- yogurt (Greek, fat-free)
- yogurt (plain and fat-free)
- zucchini

Check That Store Cupboard Too!

There are a number of dry and bottled ingredients that you may not necessarily need to buy, but which you will require if you make every recipe.

These are your store cupboard goods and include seasonings, spices, dried herbs and so on – things that you will not always need to buy more of, and which are not always absolutely essential within a recipe, but which you will probably want to have in stock.

So, have a quick check for the following items before you kick off your 17-Day Slim Down.

- bay leaves
- black peppercorns in a grinder
- canola oil
- chili flakes
- chili paste
- cider vinegar
- coriander seeds
- cornflour
- cinnamon (ground)
- cumin
- dill (dried)
- herbs (mixed, dried)
- hoisin sauce
- hot pepper sauce
- mustard (Dijon)
- olive oil
- paprika
- red wine vinegar

- rice vinegar
- vegetable stock cube
- white wine vinegar
- saffron
- salt (kosher salt ideally, as this is additive-free and comes in larger grains)
- sesame oil
- soy sauce (reduced sodium)
- thyme (dried)
- vegetable stock cube
- white pepper
- white wine vinegar

Once you have checked and topped up on these handy staples, you are all set. Time to start losing weight, and loving it!

Don't forget to share your thoughts on this book by leaving a review on Amazon.com. It takes just a few seconds.

Discover Scientifically-Proven "Shortcuts" & "Hacks" to Lose Weight FASTER (With Very Little Effort)

For this month only, you can get Linda's best-selling & most popular book absolutely free – *Weight Loss Secrets You NEED to Know.*

Get Your FREE Copy Here:
TopFitnessAdvice.com/Bonus

Discover scientifically-proven tips to help you lose weight faster and easier than ever before. With this book, readers were able to improve their weight loss results and fitness levels. So, it's highly recommended that you get this book, especially while it's free!

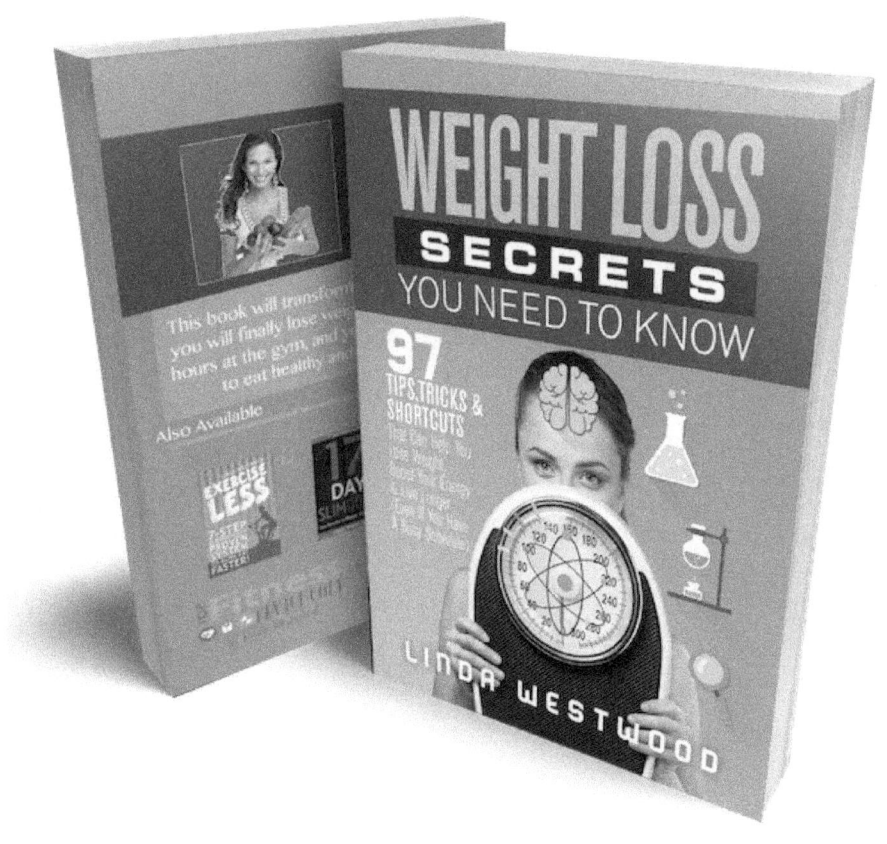

Get Your FREE Copy Here:
TopFitnessAdvice.com/Bonus

Conclusion

So, the 17 days are now up and what have you achieved? If you have followed the program correctly, you will have achieved a remarkable amount for your health and your body. You will have:

- Lost weight, which is great for your joints, heart and organs as well as helping you look fabulous.

- Have reduced your risk of heart attack, stroke, cancer, diabetes and other serious diseases.

- Slimmed inches off your body (just check that photo)!

- Upped your fiber intake so that you have aided your digestive system and cut your risk of colonic disorders and diseases.

- Help your liver and kidneys by keeping fully hydrated and going alcohol free.

- Given the quality of your skin, hair and nails a real boost.

- Become more lithe and flexible through regular exercise.

- Increased your resting metabolic rate and your energy levels.

- Worked your body to optimum levels, which means enough to tone muscles in your legs, abdomen and butt...

- ...and given a great workout to your most important muscle, your heart!

Huge kudos on creating a much healthier new you!

In less than 3 weeks, you will have transformed your body from the inside out and hopefully enjoyed the journey so far. Now, continue to enjoy these many benefits by adopting the principles of the 17-Day Slim Down and taking them forward as a far better lifestyle for you and your loved ones.

Enjoy it, whether it's for another 17 days, 17 months or, for beyond 17 more years... and for the rest of your happy, healthy life.

Final Words

I would like to thank you for purchasing my book and I hope I have been able to help you and educate you on something new.

If you have enjoyed this book and would like to share your positive thoughts, could you please take 30 seconds of your time to go back and give me a review on my Amazon book page.

I greatly appreciate seeing these reviews because it helps me share my hard work.

You can leave me a review on Amazon.com.

Again, thank you and I wish you all the best!

Enjoying this book?

Check out my other best sellers!

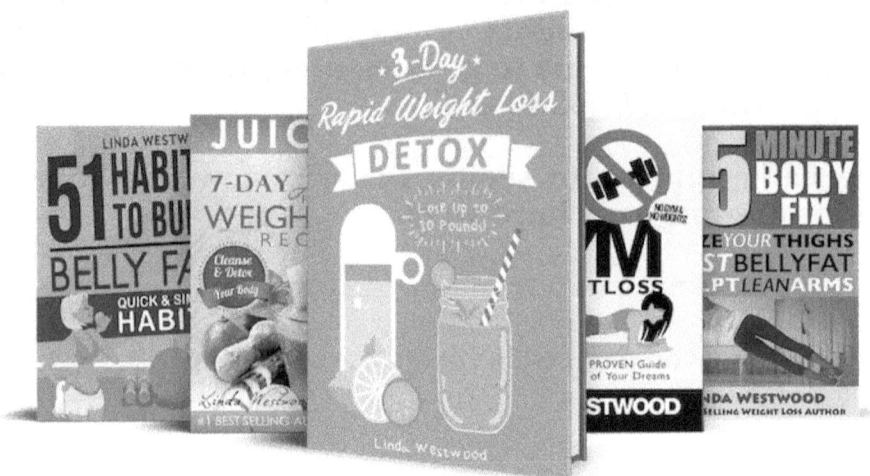

Get your next book on sale here:

TopFitnessAdvice.com/go/books

www.ingramcontent.com/pod-product-compliance
Lightning Source LLC
Chambersburg PA
CBHW031149020426
42333CB00013B/581